# MENSTRUAL CYCLE

Edited by **Olena Ivanivna Lutsenko**

**Menstrual Cycle**
http://dx.doi.org/10.5772/intechopen.76123
Edited by Olena Ivanivna Lutsenko

**Contributors**

Patricio Barriga, Sherry Stewart, Kayla Joyce, Magdalena Wiecek, Abdelhamid Benmachiche, Amel Dammene Debbih, Courtney Marsh, Rosemary Ogu, Avwebo Otoide, Preye Fiebai, Olena Ivanivna Lutsenko



First published in London, United Kingdom, 2019 by IntechOpen
IntechOpen is the global imprint of INTECHOPEN LIMITED, registered in England and Wales, registration number: 11086078, The Shard, 25th floor, 32 London Bridge Street
London, SE19SG – United Kingdom
Printed in Croatia

British Library Cataloguing-in-Publication Data
A catalogue record for this book is available from the British Library

Additional hard and PDF copies can be obtained from orders@intechopen.com

Menstrual Cycle, Edited by Olena Ivanivna Lutsenko
p. cm.
Print ISBN 978-1-78923-934-8
Online ISBN 978-1-78985-673-6
eBook (PDF) ISBN 978-1-78985-674-3

For EU product safety concerns:
IN TECH d.o.o., Prolaz Marije Krucifikse Kozulić 3, 51000 Rijeka, Croatia,
info@intechopen.com or visit our website at intechopen.com.

# Meet the editor

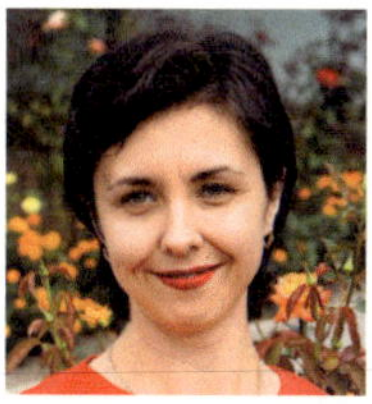

Olena Ivanivna Lutsenko studied the peculiarities of the cardiovascular system in elderly and old people for two years and received her master's degree in biology from Cherkasy National University named after Bohdan Khmelnytskyy. In 2011, she entered postgraduate studies in Cherkasy National University named after Bohdan Khmelnytskyy and began to work on the features of menstrual cycle and its relationship to hemodynamics. She now works on research topics at the Hlukhiv National Pedagogical University of Alexander Dovzhenko and teaches medical and biological disciplines. She has published over 74 scientific works including five textbooks and two monographs. Recent studies focus on women's menstrual cycle and its relationship with body typology, the period of puberty, and healthcare of the younger generation.

# Contents

# Preface

The main indicator of women's reproductive health is the menstrual cycle. Matters concerning the physiology and pathology of menstrual function have great theoretical and practical significance. The critical importance of menstrual problems includes the long course of menstrual disease, the frequent relapse of menstrual disorders, and the appearance of post-hemorrhagic anemia, which in turn leads to infertility and loss of women's ability to work.

The range of years when a woman has the ability to conceive and bear a child is called the reproductive period. This time span is closely related to the appearance of the physiological rhythm in the function of the female body, the external manifestation of which is connected to the menstrual cycle.

The menstrual cycle is a complex biological process in a woman's body: it is cyclic, its whole aim is reproduction, and it is manifested by menstrual bleeding.

By focusing on issues related to the menstrual cycle, a woman can help maintain her health and that of her future children.

In this monograph, the reader will find sections treating various questions, such as: "What is a normal menstrual cycle?", "Which features of the cardiovascular system are related to the normal menstrual cycle?", "What is menstrual syndrome?", and "What is the relationship between carrying physical loads and the menstrual cycle?" Here, scientists from around the world have presented their own research, observations, and generalizations of knowledge on the issues of menstrual cycle.

**Olena Ivanivna Lutsenko**
Department of Theory and Methods of Teaching of Natural Sciences
Hlukhiv National Pedagogical University of Alexander Dovzhenko
Ukraine

Chapter 1

# Introductory Chapter: Regulation of Ovarian-Menstrual Cycle as a Systemic Problem of Physiology of Humans

Olena Lutsenko

Additional information is available at the end of the chapter

http://dx.doi.org/10.5772/intechopen.85065

## 1. Introduction

One of the main manifestations of the vital activity of the female body is the menstrual cycle, which begins during puberty and has a rhythmic (monthly) character.

Endocrine relationships in the hypothalamic-pituitary-ovarian system are formed throughout the period of puberty. This process is regulated by certain neuroendocrine processes, which have different activities depending on age. The determinants of this regulation are the hypothalamus, pituitary gland, gonads, thyroid gland, and adrenal cortex; therefore, a certain interest is the study of the peculiarities of the formation of the hypothalamic-pituitary-ovarian hormonal system.

Back in the late nineteenth century, leading scholars D. O. Ott, S. S. Zikharev, and A. V. Reperov found that menstrual cycle is not a local process, but a wavelike reaction of the organism associated with changes in the system of the hypothalamus-pituitary-ovaries-uterus, which appears from the outside of uterine bleeding. These changes in vital processes in the body of women were called "menstrual wave" [1, 2].

So, the normal menstrual cycle is a finely coordinated cyclic process of stimulating and inhibiting effects that lead to the release of one mature egg. Various factors involved in the regulation of this process, including hormones, paracrine, and autocrine factors, are identified so far [3].

The regulation of the menstrual function passes through a complex neurohumoral path [4–6]. According to modern concepts [7–9], cyclic changes in the body of a woman are related to the implementation menstrual function and occur with the obligatory participation of five levels (or levels) of regulation. Each of them is regulated by the structures located above according to the mechanism of feedback.

The levels (links) of regulating the menstrual (reproductive) function:

1. the cerebral cortex is a cerebral structure;
2. hypothalamus-subcortical centers;
3. pituitary gland-brain application;
4. ovaries-gonads; and
5. uterus-organ-target.

Nowadays, leading scientists insist that the multilateral morphological features are closely related to the functional manifestations of sexual dimorphism [10, 11], which, in its turn, causes the sexual specificity of the processes of adaptation of the organism to external influences and, in particular, to physical activity. For women, the role of estrogen and progestogens is predominant, and for men, androgens. The degree of saturation of the body by sex hormones determines their biological effect [12–16].

Estrogens are an important link in the chain of adaptive-trophic reactions in the body [17, 18]; they have an anabolic effect but are slightly weaker than androgens, determine the degree and nature of the distribution of fatty tissue by female type, increase the growth of pelvic bones, create a female type of body proportions [19, 20], contribute to the closure of epiphyseal bone growth zones, and hinder the development of osteoporosis (resorption of bone tissue). Estrogens suppress erythropoiesis (red blood cells), reduce thrombocytopenia, promote growth of shock and minute volume of the heart, increase cardiac output, increase the volume of circulating blood, and have a positive effect on myocardial tropism and vascular tone [21, 22].

Progesterone, like estrogens, increases systolic and temporal volumes of blood and the frequency of heart contractions. Progesterone has a sodium diuretic effect and reduces the peripheral resistance of the blood vessels, which contributes to lowering blood pressure [23, 24].

Estrogens cause narrowing of the lumen of bronchioles by increasing the release of histamine and serotonin, increasing pulmonary resistance. Its direct effect increases the excitability of the respiratory center; improves the patency of bronchioles by increasing their lumen; decreases the overall pulmonary resistance; as a consequence, increases alveolar ventilation; and decreases the tone of the respiratory muscles [18, 25].

The change in the balance of steroid hormones, in particular the deficiency of progesterone and the excess of estrogens involved in the regulation of water-salt metabolism, increases reabsorption (reabsorption) of sodium in the kidneys while increasing osmotic pressure. As a result, in order to maintain homeostasis, the water is delayed in the body to compensate for the homeostasis, and, as a consequence, the body weight increases in the premenstrual and menstrual phases of the cycle. Scientists have established the influence of sex hormones on the emotional state of women [22, 26]. All of the above suggests that reproductive and exogenital functional systems are closely interrelated, and the reproductive system, in turn, has a different effect on the organs and tissues of other functional systems, which correlates the adaptation, resistance, and reactivity of the female body. In recent years, the distribution and extension theory has intensified, according to which the influence of sex steroids to one degree or another extends to the functional state of all organs and systems [10, 27, 28].

The functional state of the cardiovascular system in women has a number of features due to hormonal changes that accompany the menstrual cycle [29]. In recent years, the study of the role of estrogens and progestogens in the regulation of the function of the cardiovascular system [30].

The increased resistance of women in comparison with men to cardiovascular diseases is associated with the dynamics of cardiodynamics parameters in stressed women [23], which is determined by the sexual characteristics of the nervous and humoral regulation of the cardiovascular system. During stress, more catecholamines are released in the female body [31, 32], and their influence on the heart rhythm becomes more pronounced, but pressor responses are less prolonged than in men, which suggests that the control of the sympathetic adrenal system is more effective in the female body [33]. The factors limiting its activity include the presence of estrogens, which enhance the tone of the parasympathetic nervous system and reduce sympathetic effects on the cardiovascular system. The influence of estrogens on the vegetative level of regulation, along with their peripheral effects on the heart and blood vessels, is the basis of cardioprotective properties of estrogens. Information on the influence of androgens on the cardiovascular system and the mechanisms of its regulation are few and contradictory. Testosterone contributes to the development of hypertension and has an atherogenic effect [34]. At the same time, testosterone improves coronary blood flow in coronary arteries [35] and positively affects the mechanical function of the heart by activating the expression of heavy α chains of myosin [36]. Sexual features in cardiovascular stress reactivity are largely due to differences in the autonomic regulation of the cardiovascular system in the female and male body. Investigation of the mechanisms that determine the differences in the activity of the autonomic nervous system departments convinces in the need to study the role of sex hormones. The scarcity and contradictory nature of research data on the role of autonomic regulation of the cardiovascular system in the female and male organisms, as well as the influence of sex hormones on the autonomic balance, justify the carrying out of complex studies of the revealed phenomenon [37, 38].

Significant are the effective attempts to decipher the mechanism of the influence of sex hormones on the central nervous system that are highlighted in the works of well-known scientists [33]. The beginning of puberty is marked by a significant increase in the threshold of the sexual centers of the central nervous system (gonadostat) to steroids in the feedback system, which was first noticed by Hohlweg and Dohin (1932) and then Donovan and van der Werff Ten Bosch (1965) [38]. Further animal studies and human observation fully confirmed this assumption. The enhancement of the inhibitory effect of sex steroids on the hypothalamus has been linked with a change in the puberty of the spectrum of sex hormones—the shift in the ratio of estrogen to testosterone in favor of the latter, which is allegedly less effective in suppressing the production of gonadotropins. However, this is unlikely.

The scientific assumptions about the importance of changing the metabolism of testosterone and other androgens during puberty have been supported. So, in an experiment in many species of animals, it was discovered and demonstrated that the metabolic activity of the liver and kidneys, aimed at inactivating androgens, increases with age. Small amounts of sex hormones produced by gonads of immature animals give a more pronounced inhibitory effect due to the fact that in adult animals the inactivation of hormones is more pronounced [38]. However, this hypothesis was subjected to devastating criticism, as the androgenic effect on other target organs during puberty does not decrease but increases.

An important role in the onset of puberty may be played by not only inhibiting but also stimulating effects of sex hormones, in particular estrogens. We have convincing evidence of the leading role of estrogens in the formation of systems of the hypothalamic neurons responsible for regulating the gonadotropic function of the pituitary gland. This process begins during the period of sexual differentiation of the hypothalamus, but its final stage falls on the puberty period. It has been experimentally shown that the administration of small doses of sex hormones can cause premature puberty. Although the role of estrogens is particularly significant in the formation of pubertal in girls, however, in boys, estrogens are also an effective stimulator for secretion of gonadotropin and gonadotropins, since central nervous structures do not lose their ability to respond to the stimulating effect of estrogens during sexual differentiation [33].

During the menstrual cycle, there are significant changes in the hypothalamic-pituitary system and in the body as a whole. Cyclical changes in the structures of the hypothalamus and in the anterior lobe of the pituitary gland regulate all processes that ensure the reproductive function of the woman.

Fluctuations in mental processes and functional state during the menstrual cycle have been proven by many researchers, and the association of these oscillations with the nature of secretion of sex hormones is evident. These changes were detected in the attitude of emotional and motivational behavior [39], the electrical activity of the cerebral cortex [23, 40], the autonomic tone [41], the activity of the cerebral hemispheres [42], and the physical and mental performance [80].

However, the clear dependence of the change in the psycho-functional state, depending on the phases of the menstrual cycle, cannot be identified, and the results of the research are mainly controversial (especially concerning the premenstrual and menstrual phases). Thus, the follicular phase is considered by most researchers as a period of high mental and physical working capacity. As for the phase of ovulation, as a period of poor performance, researchers have quite controversial thoughts. At the same time, some scholars tend to believe that the menstrual cycle does not affect the psycho-functional state of the woman [43], and there are those who record a significant deterioration or improvement [26] of mental and physical performance in the premenstrual and menstrual periods.

Investigating the indicators of the functional state of the soccer players in various phases of the ovarian menstrual cycle, Buzzin VR (2009) [44] concluded that the dependence of the level of physical performance in the first phase of CMC depends mainly on the state of central hemodynamics, in stages II and V (from repolarization of the ventricles), in the IV phase (the state of the atrium), and in the III phase (from the general state of the organism). Body mass swims on the studied indicators of the body of soccer players throughout the entire biological cycle. Given that it is an integral indicator of the general state of the organism, the data obtained can be evidenced by the fact that the pursuit of football contributes to the coherence in the activity of the studied systems of the body of athletes. Perhaps, this is due to the individual nature of the body's response to the fluctuations of sex hormones during the menstrual cycle, depending on many variables of psychophysiological factors, mediating the influence of hormones on the central nervous system and higher nervous activity.

The factors that may affect the condition of women in the premenstrual phase include age, type of constitution, level of health, and typological peculiarities of higher nervous activity. Confirmation of the influence of the identified factors can be, in particular, significant differences in the level of sex hormones between people with different typological peculiarities: type of constitution [12], functional asymmetry [23], temperament [45], as well as differences between adolescent and adolescent girls [41].

The study of Naumova [71] illustrates the different effects of the phases of the ovarian-menstrual cycle on the psychomotor quality and properties of the nervous system of women. The author measured these indices during the premenstrual phase (1–3 days before menission), the menstrual phase (1–2 days), and the postmenstrual phase (1–2 days) during the 3-month period. The obtained data were compared with each other and with the background (from the beginning of menstruation on the 10th–12th day). The premenstrual phase is characterized by deterioration of psychomotor performance. Compared with the background (the period between menstruations), muscle strength and maximum frequency of movements decreased much more often than they increased. Endurance in relation to static forces varied slightly during this period and in the direction of increase [47, 48].

The menstrual phase is characterized by an increase in the muscle strength of the majority of the girls studied (but only to the background level) and the maximum frequency of movements (excess of the background level), but the endurance is somewhat reduced. At the same time, the second component of endurance attracts attention—maintaining the effort against the background of increasing fatigue [46–49]. The postmenstrual phase was accompanied by a variety of changes in the studied parameters. The maximum frequency of movements increases even more, and muscle strength and endurance are greatly reduced.

In the premenstrual phase, the mobility of the nervous processes has increased. These changes indicate an increase in the emotional and motor reactivity of women in the premenstrual phase, which corresponds to the findings of the researchers in the literature on increasing the irritability of women before menstruation [50, 51]. It is explained by the fact that thyroid gland swelling is observed in the premenstrual phase of CMC and there are symptoms of thyrotoxicosis, that is, increased production of thyroid hormones [52]. In the postmenstrual phase, the return of the neurodynamics to the background level is observed. Excitement increases, and mobility of nervous processes decreases somewhat.

The strength of the nervous system in various phases of the OMC did not undergo significant and logical changes. Consequently, as can be seen from the data presented, in different phases of the CMC, the psychomotor functions change unevenly and differently, so that the deterioration of performance on one indicator may be accompanied by an improvement in the ability to work after another [53–55]. Thus, the indicators of "external" and "internal" balances in certain phases of CMC vary in a different direction [56]. The effect of phases of the CMC on functional parameters, well-being, and mood should be taken into account in studies related to the female contingent [23, 57, 58].

The revealed neurovegetative and endocrine regularities of regulation of the ovarian-menstrual cycle are realized through individual-typological peculiarities of the hormonal status and morphology of the female body.

## 1.1 Individual features of central hemodynamics and cardiac rhythm variability in women of reproductive age

The variability of the heart rate (HRV) is a fundamental physiological property of the human body and reflects the state of regulating mechanisms, in particular the autonomic tone of the autonomic nervous system; its study contributes to the development of quality diagnosis, prognostication, and prevention of various diseases [43].

In recent years, the number of studies on the variability in the duration of the interval RR [31, 32, 34, 59, 60], blood pressure [60, 61], shock volume of blood [35, 60], respiratory arrhythmia [31, 32, 40], and communication wave changes in various hemodynamic parameters. This is due to the wide introduction of information technologies to medicine and physiology, as well as to the confirmed or highly diagnostic value of parameters of regulatory rhythms of hemodynamics.

On the adaptive-trophic role of the sympathetic department of the VNS, including in the reproduction, one of the first pointed academician Orbeli [27]. However, until now, the study of the state of the VAS, including heart rate activity, in women during the normal menstrual cycle and in the physiological and complicated pregnancy, remains insufficient. A number of review papers [43, 62] provide data on age and gender changes in some HRV indices. However, they relate mainly to short (2–5 min) records of RR intervals and performed on contingents of persons with different pathologies. At the same time, the characteristics of the wave structure of oscillation of hemodynamic indices in healthy women in different physiological conditions and loads in the ontogenesis process are insufficiently analyzed. Studies by Ketel et al. [12], conducted in randomized tubes for 149 men and 137 middle-aged women, revealed that HRV levels were inversely related to age and heart rate in both sexes. The level of LF in men is significantly higher in women than in women and is negatively related to the level of triglycerides, insulin. The power of the R-R interval for women is higher than that of men.

The widespread introduction of the ECG Holter monitoring method into the clinical practice allowed the evaluation of HRV values in the course of the day and at certain intervals and also used this method for studying the state of autonomic regulation of the cardiac rhythm [64]. Extreme values of total power of the spectrum and power in the range of very low and low frequencies in Holter monitoring of women compared to men were also recorded in Fluckiger et al. [65]. At the same time, the power in the ranges of low and high frequencies was negatively correlated with age. The total power of the spectrum decreased relatively between 20–29 years and 60–69 years by 30%.

The same gender and age characteristics of the wave structure of the cardiac rhythm were also confirmed in measurements of 302 men and 312 women conducted by Bai et al. [36], with 653 persons performed by Aubert et al. [66], and on 276 persons conducted by Barrett et al. [67]. The gender differences of HRV are measured at the sixth decade of a person's life cycle. Changes in the heart rhythm and its spectral components during orthopedic trial at this age did not have sexual differences.

There are significant differences in the reactivity of fluctuations in the duration of the R-R interval and the peripheral pressure of men and women on physical, mental, and cold loads. So in studies OV Peshakova [68] shows that women under these conditions have a greater centralization of mechanisms of regulation of the cardiovascular system, and for men—an increase in the activity of the sympathetic link of the autonomic nervous system.

Many researchers [39, 69] point out that cardiovascular analysis is more appropriate to detect minor fluctuations of the VNS activity during the menstrual cycle than the use of traditional indicators such as heart rate and arterial pressure. However, the results of studies of changes in cardiac rhythm in different phases of the menstrual cycle are still controversial. It should be noted that significant changes in HRF in women of reproductive age, whether alone or in psycho-emotional stresses, may be due to the ovarian cycle [70]. SDNN in young women was highest during the follicular phase of the menstrual cycle [26]. According to Kravchenko and co-authors [71] in women during the luteal phase compared with the follicular showed an increase in the activity of the sympathetic department of the autonomic autonomy of the autonomy according to the HRV indices. However, a group of researchers Grossman et al. [70] insists on the absence of differences in the parameters of the wave structure of blood pressure and heart rate when performing orthopedic and stimulating carotid sinus in women in different phases of the ovarian cycle.

Japanese scientists [39] demonstrate a significant increase in sympathetic and decreased parasympathetic activity in the luteal phase compared to follicular, as evidenced by an increase in LF/HF and LF values, as well as a decrease in HF in the luteal phase. The facts of the increase in the level of LF/HF in the early and middle luteal phase are presented in Hirshoren et al. [72], with the late lutein phase showing a tendency to decrease the level of LF/HF. At the same time, some researchers, Princi et al. [69] and Sato et al. [39], refute this assumption, indicating that there is no significant change. Although some researchers point to an increase in the level of HF in the follicular phase compared with the luteal and menstrual phase, measurements were made only one [15] or twice a week [73] during the cycle. Since hormonal and physiological changes during the menstrual cycle are complex, they cannot be characterized by two measurements, indicating the need for long-term research.

In studies [45], with ten completely healthy women, it was found that spontaneous baroreceptor sensitivity increases during the luteal phase compared to the follicular phase. It was stated that there were certain differences in the logRSA fluctuations during the menstrual cycle, which were related to the average NSC indices.

According to Fleischman [28], there are significant changes in both the wave structure of the cardiac rhythm and its reactivity to the burden on women in the first 20 weeks of pregnancy. So, normally in this period, the power of OT components increases, and often the synchronization of respiratory and baroreflector waves is observed. In pathological development of pregnancy, there is an inversion of such regulatory relations.

The variability of the cardiac rhythm during the physiological course of pregnancy is reduced, which indicates an increase in the activity of the sympathetic department of the autonomic nervous system [12, 13]. In women with gestosis, HRV is more pronounced. Revealed by scientists the facts of changes in HRV with other hypertensive states in pregnant women, as well as in normal and complicated childbirth, are few and controversial. The emphasis is on the prospect of further study of sympathetic activity in relation to the change in HRV in pregnant and childbearing women, as well as on the need for widespread introduction of cardiointervalography in obstetrics.

Many scientists [13, 64, 74] note that in the second and third trimesters of pregnancy, the activity of the VNS is higher (by characteristics of the wave structure of the cardiac rhythm) than in nonpregnant women. The analysis of these works shows that the decrease in HRV during pregnancy is manifested in the reduction of the values of the mathematical expectation, the mod, the mean square deviation, the variational magnitude, the variation coefficient, the power of the OT waves, the normalized power of the OT waves, and the pHN50, as well as in the increase of the amplitude of the mod, index voltage, autonomic equilibrium index, LF wavelengths, normalized LF wavelengths, VLF wavelengths, and LF/HF ratios.

At the same time, it should be noted that until now scientists have not agreed on the change in HRV at the beginning of pregnancy. Thus, Vae et al. [36] investigated that in the first trimester the HRV increases and in the second and third trimesters it decreases. According to other scholars [45, 63], HRV progressively decreases, starting with the first trimester. According to Klinkenberg et al. [75], HRV in the first trimester remains unchanged. The question remains as to the nature of the changes in BCR before delivery: according to some data [64], it increases and it contributes to the normal course of labor, and for the other [1, 13]—does not change.

The reasons for increasing the excitability of VNS during pregnancy are still not studied. Some scientists believe that increased activity occurs under the influence of chronic stress, which is considered pregnancy; others regard it as a compensation in response to systemic vasodilatation, which occurs under the influence of NO, whose production will increase significantly in pregnancy. According to Klinkenberg et al. [75], the increase in VNS activity during pregnancy is the result of a true increase in the activity of higher sympathetic centers under the influence of changes in the production of various hormones during pregnancy, as well as the result of an increase in the effectiveness of b-adrenergic effects on the heart (or a decrease in the effectiveness of M-cholinergic effects). The latter is due to an increase in the content of endogenous b-adrenergic agonists (b-AP) and endogenous b-AP sensitizers or endogenous M-cholinoreceptor blockers (M-HRP) in the blood. Previously, it was shown that in pregnancy, indeed, the content in the blood b-AP increases, while the content of M-HRP does not change. Most likely, in general, the increase in sympathetic activity is a manifestation of adaptation to pregnancy and is aimed at the formation of mechanisms that ensure the growth and development of the fetus, including inhibition of contractile activity of the uterus, increased pumping function of the heart, and gas transport function of the blood.

Studying the health of women during menopause is of great interest, both for practitioners and for theoretical scholars. This is a separate branch of health care that is socially important in all countries of the world, because in connection with the prolongation of life expectancy, the number of women over 50 years old has increased threefold [76, 77], and more than one-third of her life, a woman holds in postmenopausal care [78].

To date, some research on HSR has been devoted to the study of this phenomenon in women engaged in physical exercise and sports. Thus, the specific features of the female body and its response to intensive, often extreme, training and competitive loads, characteristic of certain sports, are rather negligible. It is believed that this circumstance does not allow to accurately formulate the extent of the impact of occupations on various sports and the desire for the highest sports results in the condition of the female body [60, 79]. However, in the HSR studies on women-tongue-men in comparison with the group of men of masters of sports and masters of the international class, it was found that men had more frequencies of HRV, in particular TP, VLF, LF, LF/HF but less HF and HF percentage (%). Thus, we see that the women of single fighters in comparison with men are noticeable strengthening of the sympathetic link of the VNS.

In the study of the variability of the heart rate in the mode of the training day in the gymnasts, it was established that the relationship between the cardiovascular system and the degree of centralization in the management of cardiac rhythm not only is preserved but also varies. At the same time, the dynamics of integral indicators of the functional state of the circulatory system in gymnasiums is rather informative for the assessment of "urgent" training effect [31, 32].

It should be noted that many researchers point out that the athlete's affiliation with a particular sports specialization determines his "vegetative portrait," which is related to the nature of the exercise, which can be offset by gender differences in HRD [78].

## Author details

Olena Lutsenko

Address all correspondence to: olena85lutsenko@gmail.com

Department of Theory and Methods of Teaching of Natural Sciences, Hlukhiv National Pedagogical University of Alexander Dovzhenko, Ukraine

## References

[1] Bleil ME, Appelhans BM, Adler NE. Pubertal timing, androgens, and obesity phenotypes in women at midlife. Clinics in Endocrinology and Metabolism. 2012;**97**:1948-1952

[2] Lemanska YA. Indicators of cardiac rhythm variability in pregnant women with cardiac arrhythmias according to Holter monitoring. Bulletin of the Institute of Obstetrics and Gynecology. 2007;**3**:15-16

[3] Bazhenova EA, Voronin IM. Evaluation of polysomnographic and hemodynamic indices in healthy girls with daily profile dipper and non dipper. Vesna, Journal of Tambov State University. 2009;**14**(1):33-36

[4] Collins P, Rosano G, Jiang C. Cardiovascular protection by oestrogen-a calcium antagonist effect? The Lancet. 1993;**341**:1264-1265

[5] Collins P. Vascular aspects of oestrogen. Journal of the Climacteric and Postmenopause. 1996;**23**:217-226

[6] Cooke WN. Head rotation during upright tilt increases cardiovagal baroreflex sensitivity. Aviation, Space, and Environmental Medicine. 2007;**78**(5):463-469

[7] Cheng Y, Cohen B, Oréa V. Baroreflex control of renal sympathetic nerve activity and spontaneous rhythms at Mayer wave's frequency in rats. Autonomic Neuroscience. 2004;**111**:80-88

[8] Kovalenko SO, Kudij LI, Lutsenko OI. Peculiarities of male and female heart rate variability. Science and Education a New Dimension. 2013;**1**(2):15

[9] Asso D. Menstruation; Menopause. Chichester, West sussex/New York; 1983. 214 p

[10] Sarafinyuk LA. Features of individual morphofunctional indices in girls with varying degrees of puberty. In: Problems, Achievements and Prospects of Development of Medical-Biological Sciences and Practical Health Care. Vol. 142. 2006. pp. 69-71

[11] Saenko VG, Chekhova VE, Gurmazhenko MO. Anatomical-physiological features of the body of women-united. In: The Repository of Luhansk National University Named after. T.G. Shevchenko. 2012. Available from: http://dspace.luguniv.edu.ua/jspui/handle/123456789/150

[12] Ketel IJ. Microvascular function has no menstrual-cycle-dependent variation in healthy ovulatory women. Microcirculation. 2009;**16**:714-724

[13] Chayka GV, Gunas IV, Mazorchuk BF. Normograms of the levels of hormones in adolescent and adolescent girls in general and different morphotypes in different phases of the menstrual cycle. Biomedical and Biosocial Anthropology. 2010;**15**:185-188

[14] Asso D. Psychological and physiological changes in severe premenstrual syndrome. Biological Psychology. 1992;**33**(2):115-132

[15] Welt CK, DJ MN, Taylor AE, Hall JE. Female reproductive aging is marked by decreased secretion of dimeric inhibin. Clinics in Endocrinology and Metabolism. 1999;**84**:105

[16] Cella F, Giordano G, Cordera R. Serum leptin concentrations during the menstrual cycle in normal-weight women: Effects of an oral triphasic estrogen-progestin medication. European journal of endocrinology. 2000;**142**(2):174-178

[17] Lichkus LG. A brief critical review of the activities of the St. Petersburg obstetric and Gynecological society during the first 25 years of its existence. Journal of Obstetrics and Women's Diseases. 1911;**3**:391-442

[18] Aubert AE, Seps B, Beckers F. Heart rate variability in athletes. Sports Medicine. 2003;**33**(12):889-919

[19] Shaparenko PP. Anthropometric and somatotypological characteristics of practically healthy urban adolescents of both sexes of the Ukrainian ethnic group. Herald Morphology. 2006;**3**(1):339-341

[20] Shepelev AE, Andriychuk VM. Comparative characteristic of somatometric parameters and indicators of harmony of physical development of girls of different medical groups. Biomedical and Biosocial Anthropology. 2012;**18**:C.117-C.120

[21] Scheer FL, Hiltona M, Mantzoros CS. Adverse metabolic and cardiovascular consequences of circadian misalignment. Proceedings of the National Academy of Sciences of the United States of America. 2009;**106**:4453-4458

[22] Wenner MM. Preserved autonomic function in amenorrheic athletes. Journal of Applied Physiology. 2006;**101**(2):590-597

[23] Shutova SV, Chichuk VN, Kopchenkina YM. Biorhythmological features of sensorimotor response in girls. Scientific Records: Series Medicine Pharmacy. 2011;**4**:35-41

[24] Cockerill IM, Cockerill JA, Wormington AM. Menstrual-cycle effects on mood and perceptual-motor performance. Journal of Psychosomatic Research. 1994;**38**(7):763-771

[25] Seebauer MS. Changes of respiratory sinus arrhythmia during the menstrual cycle depend on average heart rate. European journal of applied physiology. 2002;**87**:309-314

[26] Yamamoto M, Tsutsumi Y, Furukawa K. Influence of normal menstrual cycle on autonomic nervous activity and QT dispersion. Bioelectromagnetics. 2003;**23**:152-153

[27] Orbeli LA. Lectures on Physiology of the Nervous System; Leningrad. 1935. 328 p

[28] Tegako LI, Salivon IN. Fundamentals of Modern Anthropology; Minsk. 2010. 68 p

[29] Bosquet L, Gamelin FX, Berthoin S. Is aerobic endurance a determinant of cardiac autonomic regulation? European journal of applied physiology. 2007;**100**(3):363-369

[30] Pankova NB. Analysis of rhythm variability and arterial pressure in various functional tests in women and men. Human Physiology. 2008;**34**(4):64-72

[31] Yabluchansky NI. Fundamentals of Practical Application of Non-Invasive Technology for the Study of Human Regulatory Systems; Kharkiv. 2000. 88 p

[32] Angela R, Gregg P, Pierson A. Ovarian antral folliculogenesis during the human menstrual cycle. Human Reproduction Update. 2012;**18**(1):73-91

[33] Babichev VN. Effect of estrogens on the central nervous system. Bulletin of the Russian Academy of Medical Science. 2005;**6**:45-54

[34] Celeste NT, Mickiewicz AL. The role of the ventral pallidum in psychiatric disorders psychiatric disorders. Neuropsychopharmacology. 2010;**35**(1):337

[35] Brown SJ. The effect a respiratory acidosis on human heart rate variability. Advances in Experimental Medicine and Biology. 2008;**605**:361-365

[36] Baker FC. Circadian rhythms, sleep and the menstrual cycle. Sleep Medicine. 2007;**8**(6):613-622

[37] Barrett CJ, Guild SJ, Maipas SC. Baroreceptor denervation prevents sympathoinhibition during angiotensin II—Induced hypertension. Hypertension. 2005;**46**:168

[38] Elghozi JL. Short-term variability of blood pressure: Physiology and pharmacology. Annales Pharmaceutiques Françaises. 2008;**660**(3):158-168

[39] Siepka SM, Yoo SH, Lee C. Genetics and neurobiology of circadian clocks in mammals. Cold Spring Harbor Symposia on Quantitative Biology. 2007;**72**:251-259

[40] Bolova AA. Forecasting of Peculiarities of Sexual Development of Girls on the Basis of Vegetative Regulation Estimation: Author's Abstract. dis for the Sciences. Degree Candidate Honey. Sciences Moscow; 2009. 20 p

[41] Donovan T, Bosch SS. Physiology of Puberty. London: Edward Arnold Ltd.; 1965

[42] Lutsenko OI. Morphological factors influence on young women arterial pressure levels. Clinical Practice. 2017;**14**(5):334-337

[43] Yabluchansky NI. Variability of the Heart Rate to Assist the Practitioner For True Doctors; Kharkiv. 2010. 131 p

[44] Hinojosa-Laborde C, Chapa I, Haywood JR. Gender differences in sympathetic nervous system regulation. Clinical and Experimental Pharmacology & Physiology. 1999;**26**:122-126

[45] Lewandowski J. Sex hormone modulation of neuropeptide Y and cardiovascular responses to stress in humans. Stress: Molecular Genetic and Neurobiological Advances. 1996;**2**:569-578

[46] Chapuis B, Vidal-Petiot E, Oréa V. Linear modelling analysis of baroreflex control of arterial pressure variability in rats. The Journal of physiology. 2004;**559**:639-649

[47] Bulavenko OV, Levkivska IG. Correlation of echometric parameters of genital organs in different phases of the menstrual cycle with anthroposotometric indices of healthy girls with mesomorphic somatotype. Biomedical and Biosocial Anthropology. 2010;**15**:154-158

[48] Karsch FJ, Dierschke DJ. Sexual differentiation of pituitary function: Apparent difference between primates and rodents. Science. 1973;**179**(2):484-486

[49] Leicht AS, Hirning DA, Allen DA. Heart rate variability and endogenous sex hormones during the menstrual cycle in young women. Experimental Physiology. 2003;**94**(6):441-446

[50] Kravchenko VI. Features of regulation of cardiac rhythm during mental load in women in different phases of the menstrual cycle. Cherkasy University Bulletin: Biological Sciences Series. 2008;**128**:78-87

[51] Hottenrott K. Heart rate variability and physical exercise. Current status. Herz. 2006;**31**(6):544-552

[52] Klinkenberg AV. Heart rate variability changes in pregnant and non-pregnant women during standardized psychosocial stress. Acta obstetricia et gynecologica Scandinavica. 2009;**88**:77-82

[53] McKinley PS. The impact of menstrual cycle phase on cardiac autonomic regulation. Psychophysiology. 2009;**46**:904-1011

[54] To the doctrine of the "monthly" [Text]: diss.—Zhikharev H/SS. Spb: S. Petersburg lips type, 1896. VI, 320 p; il—(Senior doctoral dissertations admitted to protection at the Imperial War) Medical Academy in 1895-1896, No. 60, 63 p

[55] Anokhin PK. The objective reflex as an object of physiological analysis. Magazine of Higher Nervous Activity. 1962;**126**:7-21

[56] Hirshoren N. Menstrual cycle effects on the neurohumoral and autonomic nervous systems regulating the cardiovascular system. Clinics in Endocrinology and Metabolism. 2002;**87**(4):1569-1575

[57] Vasilyeva VV. Mechanisms for the formation and functioning of reproductive dominant in spontaneous and stimulated cycles. Human Physiology. 2010;**3**:55-65

[58] Sato N, Miyake S. Cardiovascular reactivity to mental stress: Relationship with menstrual cycle and gender. Journal of Physiological Anthropology and Applied Human Science. 2004;**23**:215-223

[59] Bouteau N, Tavernier B. Stroke volume variation as an indicator of fluid responsiveness. Anesthesia and Analgesia. 2004;**98**(1):278-279

[60] MacNaughton J, Banah M, McCloud P. Age related changes in follicle stimulating hormone, luteinizing hormone, oestradiol and immunoreactive inhibin in women of reproductive age. Clinical Endocrinology. 2008;**36**:339-345

[61] Fluckiger L. Differential effects of aging on heart rate variability and blood pressure variability. The Journal of Gerontology: Biological Sciences. 1999;**54**(5):219-224

[62] Moroz VM, Gunas IV, Sarafinuk LA. Age and gender characteristics of the indicators of central humor in girls and boys of adolescence. Biomedical and Biosocial Anthropology. 2008;**10**:92-97

[63] Kuczmierczyk AR. Autonomic arousal and pain sensitivity in women with premenstrual syndrome at different phases of the menstrual cycle. Journal of Psychosomatic Research. 1986;**30**(4):421-428

[64] Balgir RS. Morphological and regional variations in body dimensions of the Gujjars of different localities in North-Western India. Anthropologischer Anzeiger. 2003;**61**(3):275-285

[65] Grossman P, Taylor EW. Toward understanding respiratory sinus arrhythmia: Relations to cardiac vagal tone, evolution and biobehavioral functions. Biological Psychology. 2007;**74**(2):263-285

[66] Bai X. Influence of the menstrual cycle on nonlinear properties of heart rate variability in young women. American Journal of Physiology-Heart and Circulatory Physiology. 2009;**297**(2):765-774

[67] Biro FM, Greenspan LC, Galvez MP. Puberty in girls of the 21st century. Pediatric and Adolescent Gynecology. 2012;**25**(5):289-294

[68] Brunt VE. Short-term administration of progesterone and estradiol independently alter carotid-vasomotor, but not carotid-cardiac, baroreflex function in young women. American Journal of Physiology-Heart and Circulatory Physiology. 2013;**305**:1041-1049

[69] Rilling JK. A potential role for oxytocin in the intergenerational transmission of secure attachment. Neuropsychopharmacology. 2009;**34**(13):2621-2622

[70] Budzin VR. Features of the relationship between the indicators of the functional state of the soccer players in different phases of a specific biological cycle. Pedagogics, Psychology, Medical-Biological Problems of Physical Training and Sports. 2009;**5**:29-32

[71] Naumova VA. The influence of the ovarian-menstrual cycle on motor qualities and neurodynamics of female athletes. In: Psychophysiological Issues of Studying the Personality of the Athlete; Lviv. 1976. pp. 124-131

[72] Purdon SE. Menstrual effects on asymmetrical olfactory acuity. Journal of the International Neuropsychological Society. 2001;**7, 6**:703-709

[73] Korkushko OV, Pisaruk AV, Shatilo VB, Lishnevskaya YV, Chebotarev ND, Pogoretsky YN. Analysis of Cardiac Rhythm Variability in Clinical Practice: Age Aspects; Kyiv. 2002. 192 p

[74] Cohen B, Martinelli GP, Raphan T. The vasovagal response of the rat: Its relation to the vestibulosympathetic reflex and to Mayer waves. The FASEB Journal. 2013;**27**(7):2564-2572

[75] Lawrence JE, Ray CA, Carter JR. Vestibulosympathetic reflex during the early follicular and midluteal phases of the menstrual cycle. American Journal of Physiology-Endocrinology and Metabolism. 2008;**20**:1046-1050

[76] Malhotra A. Effects of sex hormones on development of physiological and pathological hypertrophy in male and female rats. American Journal of Physiology. 1990;**259**:866-871

[77] Princi TS. Parametric evaluation of heart rate variability during the menstrual cycle in young women. Biomedical Sciences Instrumentation. 2005;**41**:340-345

[78] Kovalenko SO, Lutsenko OI. Blood pressure and hemodynamics: Mayer waves in different phases of ovarian and menstrual cycle in women. Physiological Research. 2017;**66**:235-240

[79] Lazzaro SC, Rutledge RB, Burghart DR, Glimcher PW. The impact of menstrual cycle phase on economic choice and rationality. PLoS One. 2016;**11**(1):e0144080. DOI: 10.1371/journal.pone.0144080

[80] Veldhuijzen van Zanten JJ. Mental stress-induced haemoconcentration in women: Effects of menstrual cycle phase. Health Psychology. 2009:805-816

Chapter 2

# Normal Menstrual Cycle

Barriga-Pooley Patricio and Brantes-Glavic Sergio

Additional information is available at the end of the chapter

http://dx.doi.org/10.5772/intechopen.79876

**Abstract**

Normal menstrual cycle represents a coordinated serial event, repeated month by month, at regular intervals, in which the hypothalamus participates along with the secretion of GnRH, the pituitary gland secreting follicle stimulating hormone and luteinizing hormone (LH), and the ovary which responds to those hormones, recruiting a dominant follicle and secreting estradiol and inhibin A. Estradiol stimulates endometrial proliferation and production of cervix mucus. A peak of estradiol triggers discharge of LH, responsible for ovulation and posterior secretion of progesterone by the corpus luteum, which in turn, involutionates 14 days later if it does not receive the stimulation of hCG (pregnancy). Normal menstrual cycles last 28 ± 7 days, being accepted a fluctuation of ±2 days in the same woman, as a normal pattern, what is described as a regular cycle. Normality of these events would allow to achieve a successful embrionary implantation in the case of looking for pregnancy. For this it is required that an adequate ovule to be fertilized is reached by a capacitated spermatozoon, during the ovulatory stage. Spermatozoon can survive as long as 5 days at feminine genital tractum, but the ovum is possible to be fecundated only during 12–24 hours. Fecundation occurs at the distal third of the fallopian tube and the fecundated zygote arrives in the state of a morula, to be implanted at the endometrium 4 days later. Once the state of blastocyst is reached, it is detached from its shaggy area (hatching) and it is implanted in a receptive endometrium when the window of implantation is open (days 7–9) postovulation. The first marker of pregnancy is the detection in maternal blood of β-hCG. No more than the 25% of fertile couples exposed to pregnancy can achieve gestation at the month of exposure.

**Keywords:** menstrual cycle, fertility, concepcional cycle

## 1. Definition of normality

Menstrual cycle lasts 28 ± 7 days. Just a third of patients have cycles every 28 days and 82% fluctuations among 22 and 32 days [1].

A cycle is known as regular when the frequency has a variation of no more than 2 days. The lasting of each cycle is calculated since the first day of menstruation until the previous day of next menstruation. The cycle frequency is regulated by the hypothalamus-pituitary-gonadal axis; hormones such as follicle stimulating hormone (FSH) and luteinizing hormone (LH) must reach their effectors at the ovarian level where a dominant follicle must be recruited and developed, secrete estradiol, in enough amounts to obtain endometrial receptivity but also participating directly in a feedback-regulated control of the cycle.

Cycles show more irregularity in the extremes of the reproductive lifespan, during the first 2 years from the menarche and during the perimenopausal transition. The ovarian cycle has two stages separated by ovulation, the first, from the beginning of the cycle to ovulation, is called the follicular or proliferative phase. The second, between ovulation and the next menstruation, is called the luteal phase or secretory phase.

The follicular phase is characterized by the maturation of the follicle containing an ovule and a retinue of follicular cells, which are responsible for transforming androstenedione into estradiol, which in turn is released and, among many other actions, stimulates endometrial renewal.

The luteal phase, named because the follicular cavity that left the ovule after hatching, is transformed into a corpus luteum and continues to produce estrogen, but it also releases important amounts of progesterone. The luteal phase is preceded by a significant increase in LH, and ovulation marks its onset; then, it lasts ±14 fairly constant days when comparing different women. During this phase, the average total body temperature of women is constantly 0.5°C higher than in the follicular phase.

If there is no embryo implantation, the endometrium is detached giving rise to menstrual flow, which has normal volume parameters, up to 80 mL, in duration, 3–8 days, content, absence of clots and symptoms, and absence of pain.

It is considered that the conserved cyclicity expresses that the hypothalamic-pituitary-gonadal axis is healthy. The ovaries do not alternate to ovulate.

## 2. Important concepts

**Ovarian reserve**: *it corresponds to the number of follicles that a woman has and it is defined during fetal life and then the number of follicles goes slowing down gradually.*

When is born, each woman counts with a fixed number of ova, which are getting lost with the past of years (atresia) Delaying maternity is nonrecommendable, since at higher age the risk of not having ovum of a good quality at the moment when a pregnancy is planned.

In a woman fertility, among 38–40 years is lower than at 25–30 years. Atresia of oocytes is a continuous process that never stops not even with the use of anovulatory or pregnancy.

**Oocyte atresia:** *it is the mechanism of follicular apoptosis that seems to contribute to the selection of optimal ovules.* During the early fetal stage, about 7,000,000 oocytes are formed in the ovary.

http://dx.doi.org/10.5772/intechopen.79876

Before birth, the ovular reserve has been reduced to one-third by mechanisms of apoptosis (programmed death).

At birth, only 1–2 million oocytes remain in the ovary and during puberty, there are usually 300,000 available for eventual ovulation. In fact, they will only ovulate between 400 and 500 throughout the lifespan. Then, through the female reproductive life, between the periods of puberty and menopause, about 250,000 follicles will be destined to die, reaching less than 1000 during perimenopause (**Figure 1**).

**Sex steroids—estrogens and progesterone:** Estrogens are steroid hormones produced by the granulosa follicle, the corpus luteum, and the placenta (if there is pregnancy). Its synthesis comes from cholesterol molecules. Progesterone is synthetized by corpus luteum and placenta, if there is pregnancy.

Of the estrogens, the most potent is estradiol. The actions they develop are:

- *Female genital apparatus*: they stimulate the growth and development of the female sexual organs and the proliferation of the endometrium during the sexual cycle.
- *Breast*: they favor the growth of the mammary ducts and are, in part, responsible for the development of the mammary gland during puberty.
- *Bone*: they regulate the osteoclastic activity and stimulate the osteoblastic activity, in such a way that they are essential to maintain adequate bone mineralization.

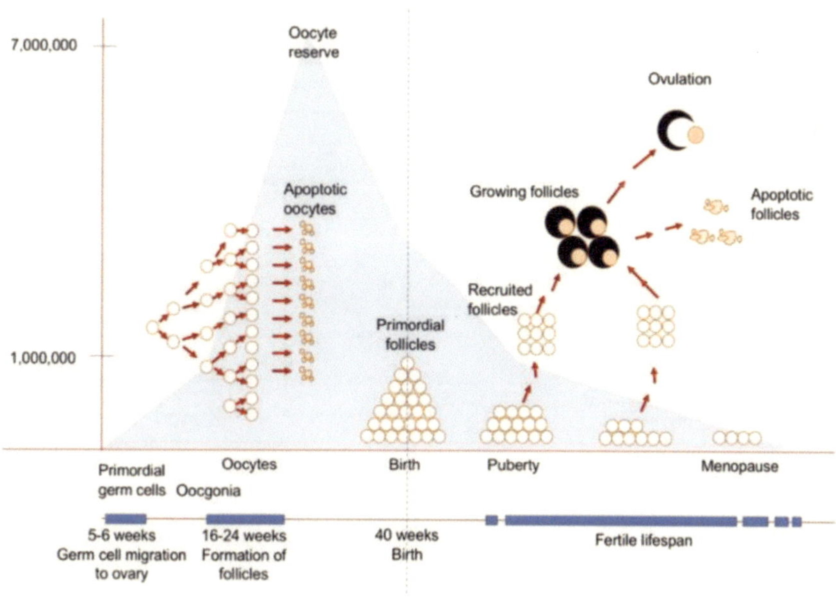


**Figure 1.** The number of oocytes in any woman comes defined at the moment of birth and slow down inevitably during her life during her life from 1 to 2 million at the moment of birth at 300,000 to go decreasing through her life 25,000 at 37–38 years and near 500 during the postmenopause.

- *Cardiometabolic*: estrogen relaxes the smooth muscle of arterioles, increases HDL cholesterol, and lowers LDL cholesterol, which has been associated with the lower incidence of cardiovascular disease that women have in relation to men, especially before menopause.

Progesterone is also a steroid hormone. It is responsible for the progestational changes of the endometrium. On the breasts, progesterone stimulates the development of the lobes, being its action complementary to that of the estrogens. Progesterone is thermogenic and contributes to the increase in basal temperature experienced by some women after ovulation.

## 3. Follicular phase

Follicular phase begins the very first day of menstruation. The development of ovarian follicles, named folliculogenesis, begins at the last days of menstrual cycle before the release of mature follicle during ovulation (**Figure 2**).

When a pregnancy did not occur, the release of inhibin A and sex steroids are reduced by the end of the functional period of the corpus luteum. Both falls contribute to reduce the release of FSH by feedback at the central level, which is dependent on pulsatility of hypothalamic GnRH. This is how FSH increases during the last days of the menstrual cycle (**Figures 3** and **4**) [2].

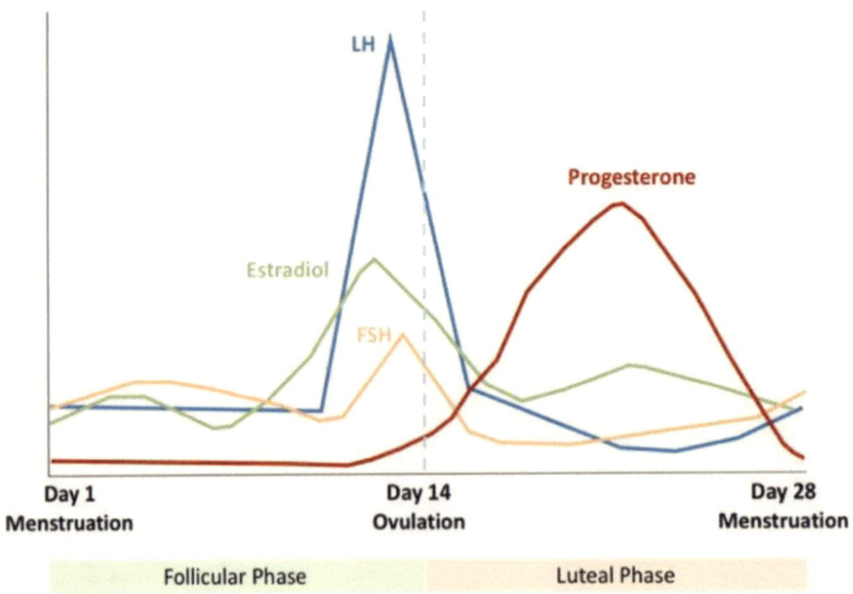


**Figure 2.** The menstrual cycle has two phases, follicular phase and luteal phase. The follicular phase begins with menstruation. The follicle stimulating hormone (FSH) increases released by the anterior pituitary gland and stimulates follicular growth and estradiol production. The 17 beta-estradiol produced by the follicles exerts negative feedback on the FSH. Estradiol continues to increase due to the growth of the dominant follicle. The LH increases sharply to trigger ovulation. Immediately after ovulation, the luteal phase begins. The corpus luteum produces progesterone and 17 beta-estradiol concentrations of progesterone and estradiol decrease, menstruation begins a new cycle, unless a pregnancy has been established.

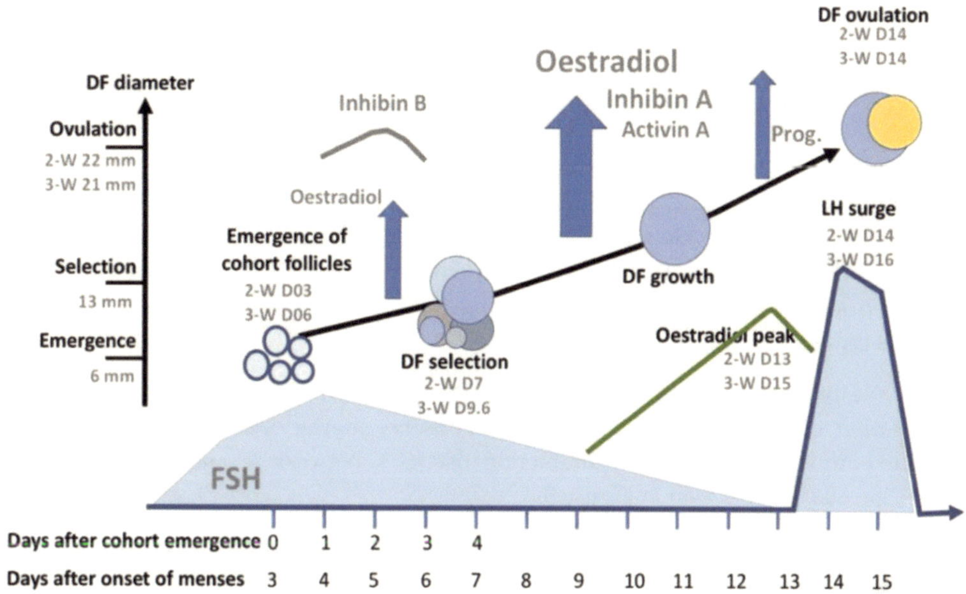


**Figure 3.** Dynamic scheme of follicular activity and the changes in gonadotropins, steroids, and inhibins during follicular phase of menstrual cycle.

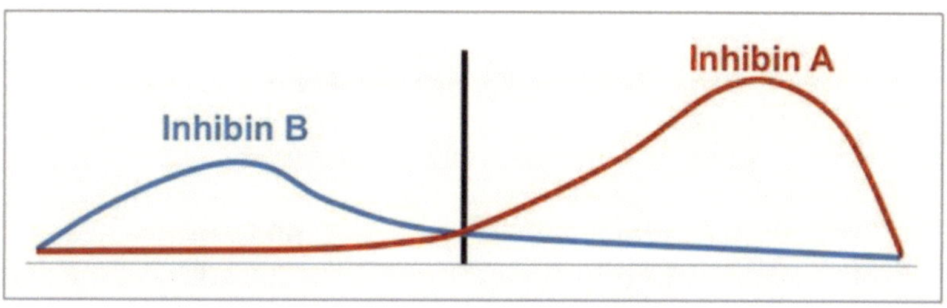


**Figure 4.** The level of inhibin changes through menstrual cycle. Inhibin B dominates follicular phase during the cycle while inhibin A dominates luteal phase.

The progressive elevation of FSH allows many follicles to be recruited simultaneously. Nevertheless, only some persist, in such a way that an approximate 99% of the cycles, only a dominant follicle will be destined to ovulate, during the next menstrual cycle.

The remaining 1% has codominance, that is two dominant follicles, which eventually can generate a double ovulation at the risk of a multiple pregnancy.

In women from 19 to 42 years, follicular phase has an average duration of 14.6 days, however, to be precise on each woman in what step of the cycle she is very difficult because of the following reasons:

- Duration of menstrual cycle is very changing, even among young women of similar ages, with variations described from 25 to 34 days.

- Changes that normally occur during the fertile lifespan, between the menarche to menopause. Some women may have long and irregular cycles, many times associated to abundant uterine bleeding, at the first 2 years after to menarche and 4–6 years that precede menopause.
- Besides there is a wide range of presentation for both phases of the cycle, the follicular phase may last from 10 to 23 days and luteal phases could last between 7 and 19 days. Only 10% of women with a cycle of 28 days shows follicular and luteal phase of 14 days. The variability depends more on follicular phase, which vary ±3–7 days with time, depending on the estrogen take off (ETO), at the beginning of the middle follicular phase on each cycle, which is the main explanation for the duration of cycles.
- Finally, despite of normal length in their cycles, 7% of women of 25–39 years may show anovulation, even though is more frequent to observe shorter cycles or longer ones, especially in early postmenarche and premenopause (60% between 10 and 14 years and 34% older than 50 years) as seen in **Figure 5**.
- Other environmental, ethnic, or even socioeconomic factors may affect the duration of the cycle and bleeding.

At the development of dominant follicle (DF), three steps have been described namely, **recruiting, selection,** and **dominance** (**Figure 6**). Recruiting stage is developed during the days 1–4 of menstrual cycle.

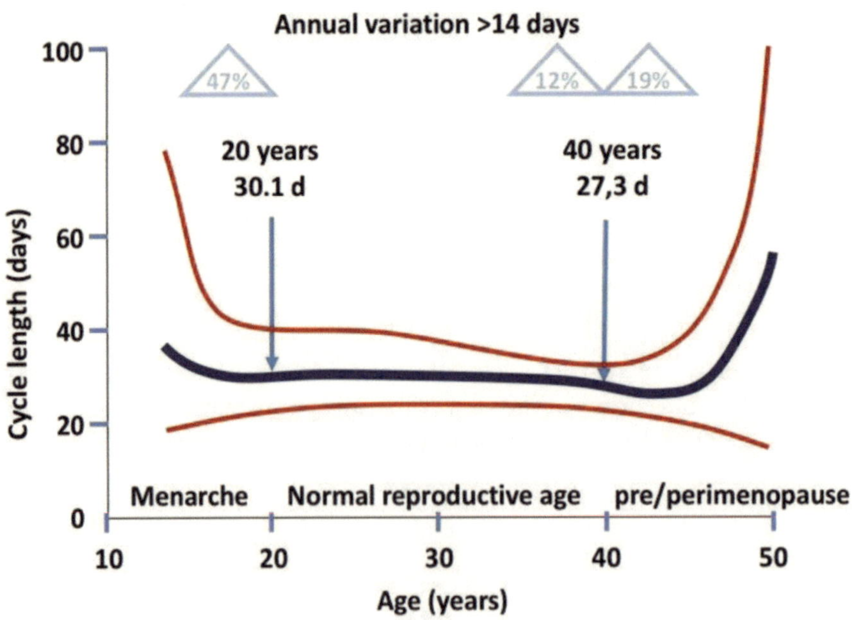


**Figure 5.** Menstrual cycle lasting variation according to age. Graphic shows the average lasting of the cycle and the range (percentiles 95 and 5) yrs. = years, d = days. Triangles indicate the group of age in the percentage of women with more than14 days of variation of a cycle during a year. From Mihm et al. [3].

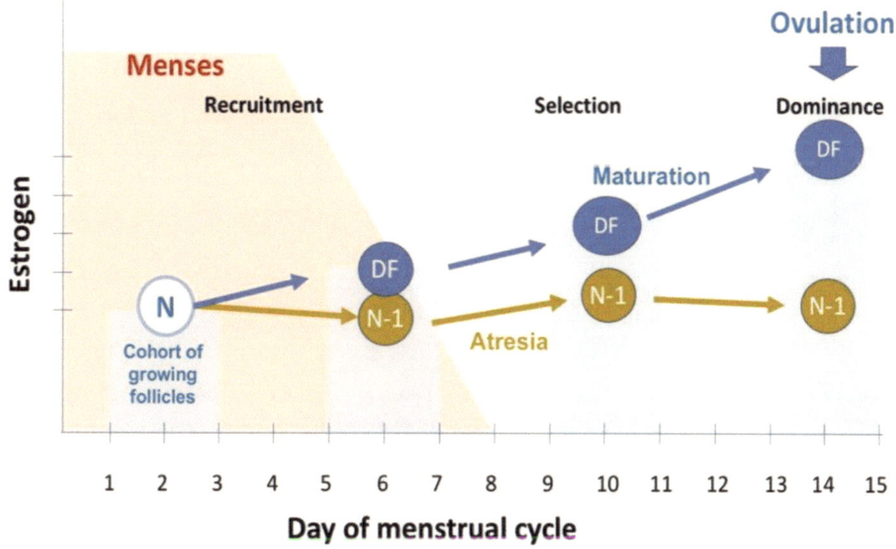


**Figure 6.** Time lapse of recruiting, selection, and ovulation of dominant follicle (DF) with the beginning of atresia in the other follicles of the group. Adapted from Hodgen [4].

During the follicular phase, FSH is responsible for recruitment among those follicles that remain available. Between days 5 and 7 of the cycle, follicular selection normally occurs, to allow only one follicle, the dominant follicle (FD) to ovulate and the rest to experience atresia. Anti-müllerian hormone (AMH), which is secreted in the granular layer, also participates in the selection of FD. On day 8 of the cycle, the FD promotes its own growth, suppressing the maturation of the other ovarian follicles.

During the follicular phase, estradiol plasma levels are higher along with the growth of the number of granulosa cells and the growth of the DF. FSH receptors are found exclusively in the cell membrane of granulosa cells. The increase in FSH during the late luteal phase induces its own FSH receptors and eventually increases the secretion of estradiol by the granulosa cells by transforming androstenedione, which diffuses from the theca cells (**Figure 7**).

It is important to point out that the increase in the numbers of receptors of FSH is due to an increase in the population of granulosa cells and not to an increase of the concentration of receptors of FSH on them. Each granulosa cell has 1500 receptors of FSH at secondary stage of follicular development, and the number of receptors of FSH stays constant during the rest of DF growing.

The increase in estradiol secretion also upregulates their own receptors, increasing the total of estradiol receptors (ER) in the granulosa cells. On the other hand, in the presence of estradiol, FSH stimulates the formation of LH receptors in the same cells, which allows the secretion of small amounts of progesterone and 17-hydroxyprogesterone (17 OHP) that would exert positive feedback on the pituitary gland. Already sensitized by the increase of estrogen, thus allowing the release of luteinizing hormone (LH) and achieve its peak. FSH also stimulates many steroidogenic enzymes such as aromatase and 3β-hydroxysteroid dehydrogenase (3β-HSD).

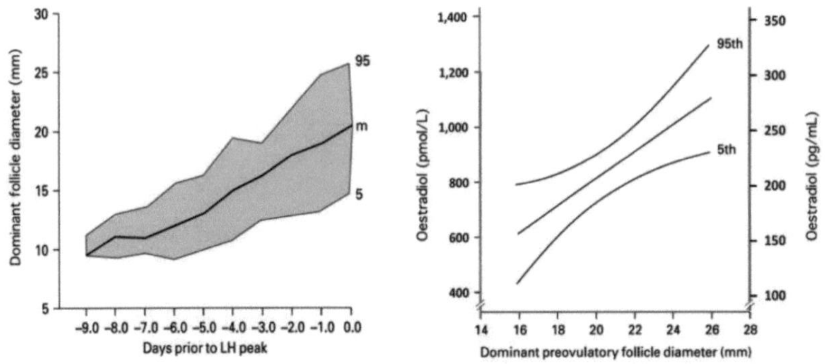


**Figure 7.** Diameter of dominant follicle (DF) days prior to LH peak and plasma concentration of estradiol per follicle diameter (curved lines are 95th and 5th percentiles). Adapted from Macklon and Fauser [5].

There are other signaling pathways that impact the differentiation of theca cells, not only LH but also insulin-like 3 (INSL3) that appear to modulate LH-mediated androgen biosynthesis and increased follicle cell apoptosis and luteal regression, bone morphogenetic proteins (BMPs) produced by granulosa cells, and/or oocytes who antagonized the effects of LH and INSL3, the circadian clock genes, androgens, and estrogens and (2) theca-associated vascular, immune and fibroblast cells, as well as the cytokines and matrix factors that play key roles in follicle growth [6].

At **Table 1**, production rates are presented for sexual steroids during follicular phase, luteal phase at the moment of ovulation.

Differently from granulose cells, LH receptors are localized at theca cells during all of the stages of menstrual cycle. LH receptors stimulates granuloma's cells. LH stimulates the production of androstenedione and at a lesser level the production of testosterone at the theca cells.

Androstenedione is then transported to the cells of granulosa where it is aromatized, and finally, it becomes estradiol 17-β-hydroxysteroid dehydrogenase type I. This is known as the

| Sex steroids* | Early follicular | Preovulatory | Mid-luteal |
|---|---|---|---|
| Progesterone (mg) | 1 | 4 | 25 |
| 17α-Hydroxyprogesterone (mg) | 0.5 | 4 | 4 |
| 17α-Hydroxyprogesterone (mg) | 7 | 7 | 7 |
| Androstenedione (mg) | 2.6 | 4.7 | 3.4 |
| Testosterone (μg) | 144 | 171 | 126 |
| Estrone (μg) | 50 | 350 | 250 |
| Estradiol (μg) | 36 | 380 | 250 |

*Values are expressed in milligrams or micrograms per 24 hours.

From Baird and Fraser [7].

**Table 1.** Production rate of sex steroids in women at different stages of the menstrual cycle.

hypothesis of two cells and two gonadotropins of the regulation of synthesis on the ovary (**Figure 8**).

The normal follicular phase has been divided in two stages: (a) early and (b) middle and (c) late, to allow a better comprehension of the endocrine events that will be finally responsible of ovulation.

**Early follicular phase (days 1–4):** it begins with the first day of menstruation. Follicular recruitment occurs due to the elevation of FSH, as a consequence of the decrease in estradiol, progesterone, and inhibin A released by the corpus luteum of the previous cycle, allowing the number of LH receptors to increase in the cells of the teak and the granulosa. The plasma levels of estradiol tend to remain low at this stage (**Figure 1**).

**Medium follicular phase (days 5–7):** as the recruitment and growth of follicles induced by FSH progress, estradiol increases slowly in a progressive manner thanks to the increased activity of CYP19, an FSH-dependent aromatase that is present in granulosa cells. The follicle that achieves the highest number of FSH receptors may aromatize more estradiol and become the dominant follicle. The other follicles, with fewer receptors for FSH, suffer atresia. For estrogen synthesis, it is necessary for the thecal cells to produce androgens, under the stimulus of LH, and for these to diffuse to the granulosa cells. Simultaneously, two glycoproteins, activin and inhibin, are produced in the theca and granulose, with local actions. Inhibin B exerts a negative hypophyseal feedback effect, where it potentiates the effect of estradiol and inhibits the synthesis and release of FSH [9, 10]. This would be a mechanism to achieve dominance giving an advantage to the follicle that has greater

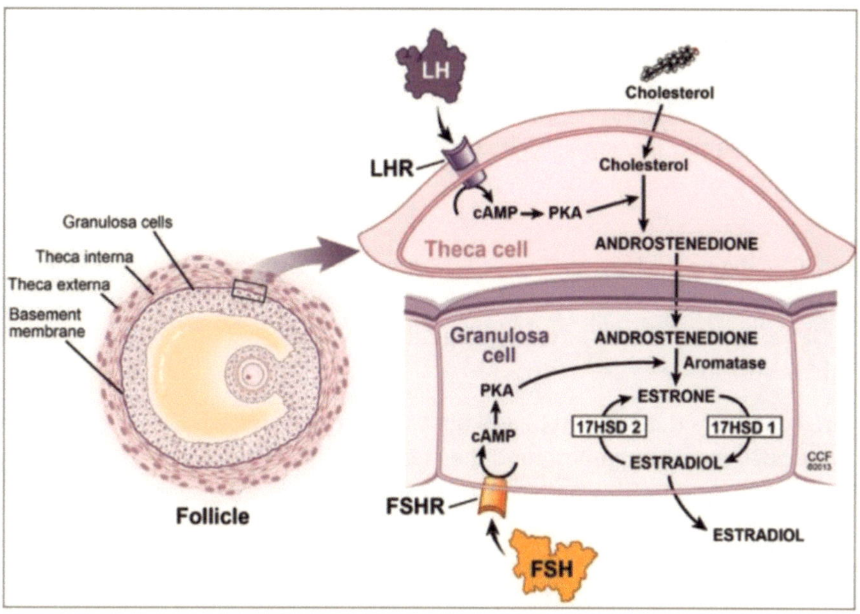


**Figure 8.** Two cells and two gonadotropins, on the regulation and the synthesis of estrogens at the ovary. From: Doshi and Agarwal [8].

development. The estrogen take-off (ETO) marks the successful establishment of the dominance of a follicle.

The FD develops its internal theca and increases receptivity to LH, which stimulates the production of androgens by degrading molecules of cholesterol to progesterone and from this to dehydroepiandrosterone, androstenedione, and testosterone.

At the end of this phase, the granulosa-theca complex of the FD has almost complete functionality to enter the late follicular phase.

**Late follicular phase (days 8–12):** this period is characterized by the elevation of estrogens that come from the DF, reaching its maximum values between 40 and 50 hours, before an elevation of FSH that precedes the ovulatory peak of LH. This preovulatory follicle reaches an average diameter of 15–20 mm.

### 3.1. Follicular phase and fertility

The moment of greatest likelihood of successful fertilization is intercourse on the day before ovulation. However, the potentially fertile period, which depends on sperm survival, can extend from 5 days before ovulation. Those pregnancies that have been obtained after day 14, are associated with later ovulation, a normal variability in the duration of the follicular phase depending on the time of the ETO.

It is believed that cycles of 30–31 days and 5 days of bleeding would have a higher probability of pregnancy [11], perhaps due to better quality of the DF, good function of the corpus luteum and optimal endometrial receptivity. The moment of the fertile window is quite variable. It has been reported that a significant number of women with regular menstrual cycles can be in their fertile window before day 10 or after day 17, of their menstrual cycle [12]. However, it seems that the possibility of pregnancy is low when the cycles are short, less than 25 days [13].

In clinical practice, to determine the fertility potential of a given cycle, indirect methods are used, which require observing at least one of the three primary signs of fertility (basal body temperature, cervical mucus and position of the cervix), known as methods based on symptoms.

There are kits to detect the increase in LH, which occurs 24–36 hours before ovulation named ovulation predictor kits (OPK). Those urine-based ovulation test kits are available in versions standard OPKs, digital OPKs or advanced digital OPKs, but some saliva-based ovulation tests are available also.

Computerized devices that interpret basal body temperature, urinary test results, or changes in saliva are called fertility monitors, and there are different types: urine-based fertility monitors, perspiration-based fertility monitors and saliva-based fertility monitors.

In the monitoring of assisted fertility procedures, effective follicular follow-up with ultrasonography is preferred.

In infertility treatments, ovulation inducers are used that increase endogenous levels of FSH or eleven therapeutically by administering FSH parenterally, which manages to rescue

http://dx.doi.org/10.5772/intechopen.79876

multiple follicles from atresia. So, this patient has a higher risk of multiple ovulation. It is interesting to note that when rescuing follicles from atresia, the follicular endowment remains the same, so that follicles will not be depleted in an accelerated manner.

### 3.2. Follicle types

At born, woman count with primordial follicles (PF), each surrounded by one layer of cells of granulosa and are detained at the pro phase of the first meiotic division.

During adolescence, the woman has antral follicles that depend on FSH. On average, this follicle takes 14 days to mature to preovulatory FD. They are derived from a recruitment process that is independent of FSH and is mainly regulated by the anti-müllerian hormone (AMH), which is produced by the granulosa cells of the follicles in early development and inhibits the transition from the primordial to the primary follicular stage [14]. AMH levels can be measured in serum and used to measure the follicular reserve (**Figures 9 and 10**).

Primordial follicles (PF) are independent of FSH. Their average life is 60–65 days, then they are transformed in to preantral follicles (PAF), also independent of FSH, and are surrounded by many layers of granulosa's cells and also by theca cells. In this process, many primordial follicles suffer atresia (**Figure 11**).

Due to the presence of 5α-reductase, the early preantral and antral follicles produce more androstenedione and testosterone compared to the estrogen rate. 5α-reductase is the enzyme responsible for converting testosterone to dihydrotestosterone (DHT). Once testosterone has been reduced by 5α, DHT cannot be aromatized.

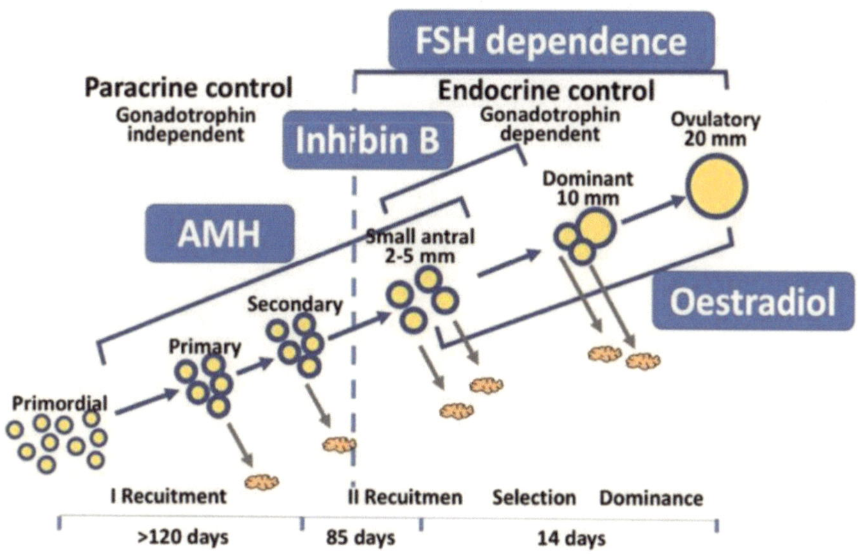


**Figure 9.** AMH is involved in the paracrine control of recruitment in the first stage, when the process is still independent of gonadotropins. AMH can not only reflect the number of early antral follicles in the process of development, but also those in earlier stages. Adapted from Ref. [1].

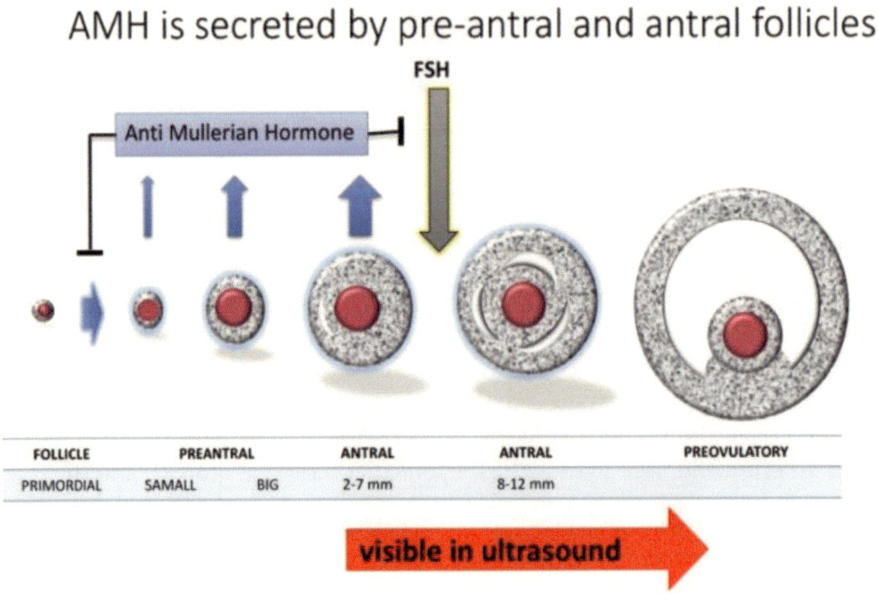


**Figure 10.** Clinical witnesses of the follicular development in stage pre- and postdependence of FSH: AMH and ultrasound, respectively. Adapted from Ref. [15].

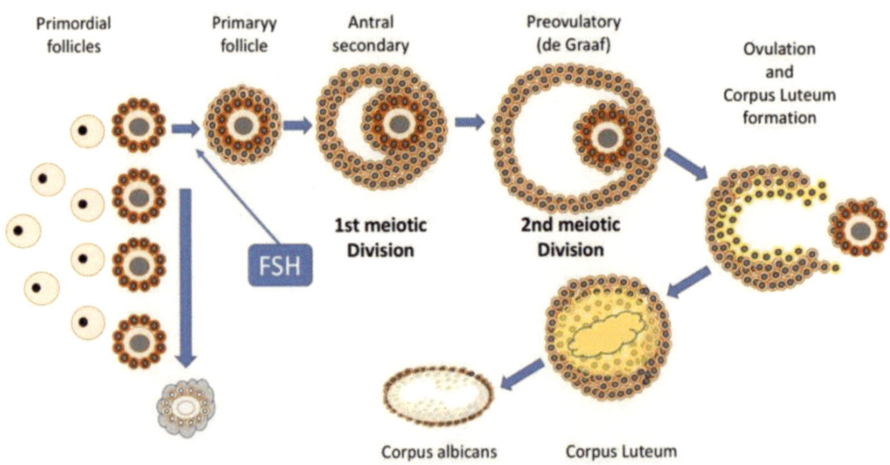


**Figure 11.** Follicular dynamics and illustration of folliculogenesis process.

With the increase in age in women, the involution of granulosa cells decreases the levels of inhibin production. Because of this, when a woman approaches menopause her FSH levels become higher, a sign that her ovarian reserve has decreased. On the other hand, the perimenopausal follicles are of the worst quality, half have chromosomal alterations.

As mentioned, the development of the preantral follicle is independent of FSH, so any follicle that grows beyond this point will require an interaction.

Secretion of gonadotropin is regulated by the releasing hormone of gonadotropin (GnRH), steroidal hormones, and diverse peptides released by dominant follicle.

Among substances that can be found al follicular liquid there are steroids, pituitary hormones, plasmatic proteins, proteoglycans, and ovarian factors nonsteroidal, which regulate the micro environment of the ovary and the steroidogenesis of the granulosa.

Factors of growing such as the insulin growth factors 1 and 2 (IGF1, IGF2) and the epidermal growth factor (EGF) would have an important role at the development and maturity of oocytes. Concentration of ovarian steroids is higher at follicular liquid compared to plasmatic concentrations.

There are two population of antral follicles: **big follicles**, which measure more than 6 mm diameter, and **little follicles**, less than 8 mm. In big follicles, concentrations of FSH are higher. Estrogen and progesterone are higher as well, while prolactin concentration is lower. Inside little follicles, prolactin and androgen levels are higher in comparison to big antral follicles.

In addition, as mentioned, FSH increases during the early follicular phase and then begins to decrease until the ovulation phase, except in the short preovulatory peak. In contrast, LH is low in the early follicular phase and begins to increase in the middle follicular phase due to positive feedback of increasing levels of estrogen.

To achieve positive feedback of LH release, plasma estradiol should be greater than 200 pg/ml, for at least 48 hours. The gonadotropins are secreted in a pulsatile manner in the anterior pituitary, with a frequency and widening of pulses that change according to the phase of the menstrual cycle (**Figure 12**).

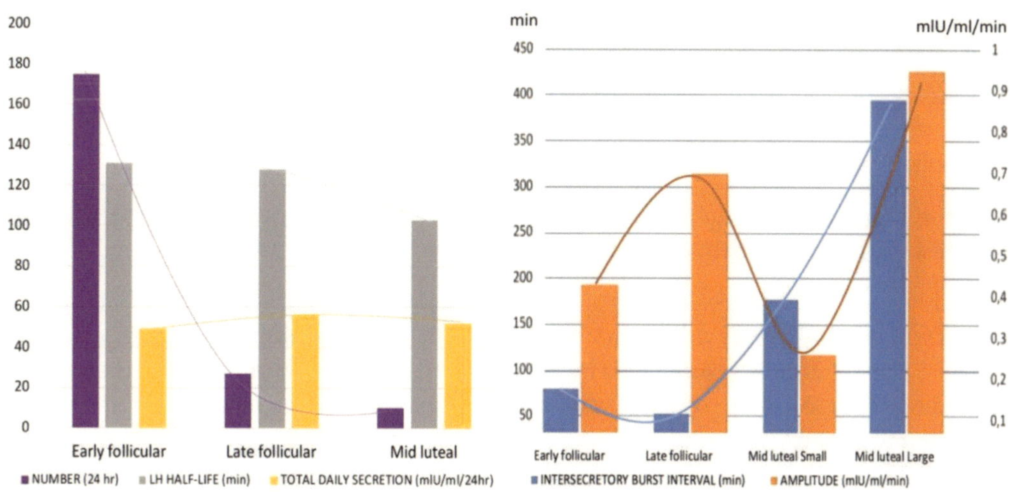


**Figure 12.** Pulses of LH throughout a normal cycle. Number of pulses per 24 h decreases, but total daily secretion and LH half-life are stable. The intersecretory burst interval becomes longer as the cycle progresses, being very long in the luteal phase, whereas the pulse amplitude of LH shows a dichotomous behavior, with small and high waves. Adapted from data of Sollenberger et al. [16].

During early follicular phase, secretion of LH occurs to a frequency of pulse from 60 to 90 minutes with a widening of pulse constant but variations on number of pulses intersecretory burst interval and pulse amplitude [16]. During late follicular phase, previous to ovulation, frequency of pulse increases and widening may be beginning to increase. Most of women have widening of pulse of LH beginning to increase after ovulation.

Once menstruation is produced, levels of FSH begin to decrease due to negative retro alimentation on inhibin B produced by developing follicle.

## 4. Ovulation

Hatching occurs 10–12 hours after peak of LH (**Figure 8**). Augmentation of LH is generated by significative raising of estradiol, with levels between 200 and 450 pg/mL, produced at the preovulatory follicle.

The critical concentration of estradiol needed to initiate positive feedback requires that the dominant follicle reach a size >15 mm in diameter. The increase in LH occurs 34–36 hours before ovulation and is a very reliable predictor of ovulation (**Figure 9**). This increase in LH is responsible for the luteinization of granulosa cells that stimulates the synthesis of progesterone and also estradiol. In addition, the LH increase resumes the second meiotic division and the chromosomal reduction in the oocyte with the release of the first polar corpuscle.

Estradiol levels decrease abruptly immediately before peak of LH. This can be due to regulation to down of LH from its own receptor or due to direct inhibition of estradiol synthesis because of progesterone.

Progesterone also participates in the stimulation of the increase in FSH in the middle of the cycle (**Figure 13**).

This increase in FSH would produce the release of oocytes from their follicular junctions, to stimulate the plasminogen activator and increase the LH receptors in the granulosa. The exact mechanism responsible for the post ovulatory fall is unknown.

Decrease in LH would occur as the consequence of the loss of positive retro alimentation of estrogens the inhibitory retro alimentation of progesterone (**Figure 14**).

It takes 36 hours from the peak of estrogen until ovulation occurs. The time to ovulation measured from the peak of LH is 12 hours; considering the time of detection in urine, ovulation will take place at 24 hours since LH is measured in the urine. The hormone hCG is similar to LH and can be used as an exogenous hormone to trigger ovulation, which will occur 36 hours after administration.

During the ovulatory period, progesterone and prostaglandins are secreted inside the follicle, as well as proteolytic enzymes. This results in digestion and rupture of the follicular wall allowing hatching, commonly called ovulation [18].

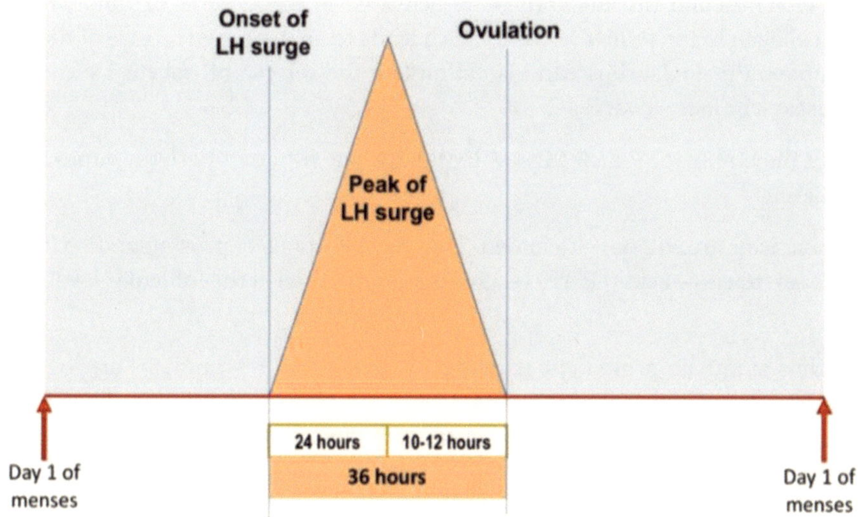


**Figure 13.** Increase of LH precedes ovulation in 36 hours. Peak, on the other side, precedes ovulation in 10–12 hours.

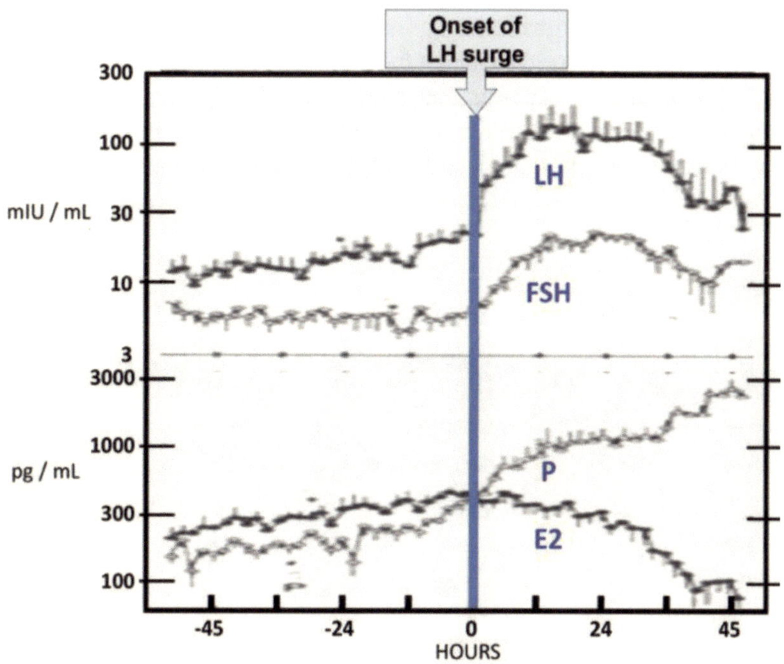


**Figure 14.** Changes in ovarian gonadotropins and steroids in the middle of the cycle, just before ovulation. The beginning of the increase of LH is at time. 0 time. Abs: E2, estrogen; P, progesterone. Adapted from Hoff et al. [17].

Proteolytic enzymes and prostaglandins are activated in response to LH and progesterone and digest collagen in the follicular wall, which leads to an explosive release of the cumulus-oocyte complex. Prostaglandins can also stimulate the release of oocytes, stimulating the smooth muscle within the ovary.

The point of the dominant follicle closest to the ovarian surface where the rupture occurs is called a "stigma."

All the mechanisms are still not elucidated. The concentrations of prostaglandins E and F and hydroxyeicosatetraenoic acid (HETE) reach a maximum level at the follicular level just before ovulation.

Prostaglandins stimulate proteolytic enzymes, whereas HETE stimulates angiogenesis and hyperemia. The use of high doses of prostaglandin inhibitors could hinder the follicular rupture, causing what is known as luteinized unruptured follicle syndrome, and can be observed in fertile and infertile women.

Consequently, it should be recommended to women in search of pregnancy and especially that with fertility problems, avoid the intake of inhibitors of prostaglandin synthesis, and inhibitors of cyclooxygenase (COX), in fact, are being investigated as an alternative to morning after pill in emergency contraception [19, 20].

For ovulation to occur, a series of complex molecular mechanisms that commence after the gonadotrophin surge must be given. These include intracellular signaling, gene regulation, and remodeling of tissue structure in each of the distinct ovarian compartments, which can be summarized in (a) ovulatory mediators that exert effects through the cumulus cell complex, (b) convergence of ovulatory signals through the cumulus complex co-ordinates the mechanistic processes that control oocyte maturation and ovulation, and (c) other multiple inputs, including

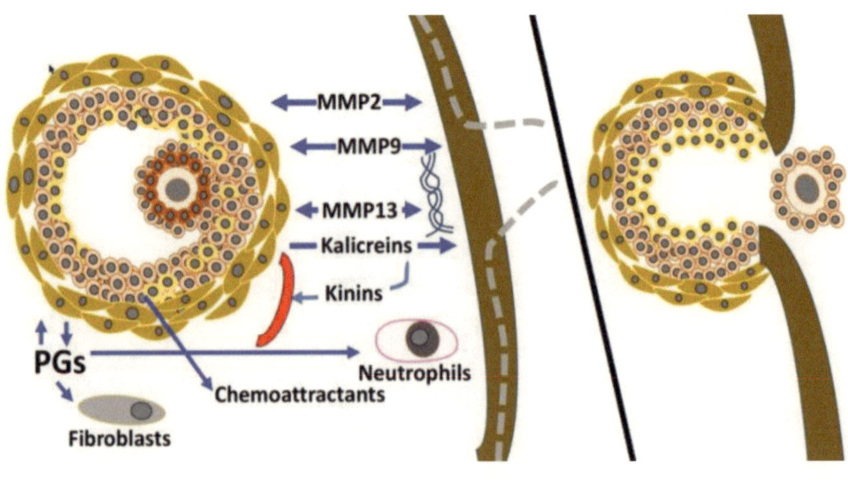


**Figure 15.** Proposed mechanisms at follicular rupture. LH stimulates the expression of genes in granulosa cells (PR, PGS-2) that control the activation of matrix metalloproteinases (MMPs), leading to the breakdown and remodeling of extracellular matrices and the surface epithelium to allow rupture of the follicle and extrusion of the oocyte (ovulation). Modified from Richards et al. [22].

endocrine hormones, immune and metabolic signals, as well as intrafollicular paracrine factors from the theca, mural and cumulus granulosa cells, and the oocyte itself. Therefore, healthy and meiotically competent oocytes and the coordination and synchronization of endocrine, paracrine, immune, and metabolic signals acting mainly through the cumulus compartment exert control on oocyte maturation, developmental, and ovulation process [21].

Mechanisms suggested implied in follicle rupture [22] are shown in **Figure 15**.

## 5. Luteal phase

This phase lasts 14 days in most women after ovulation. The granulosa cells that are not released with the oocyte acquire a vacuolated appearance and a characteristic yellow color due to the concentration of a carotenoid called lutein and the incorporation of fat drops. No other function has been described for lutein than being a powerful antioxidant.

The luteinized cells combine with the newly formed theca-lutein cells together with the surrounding stroma; thus, originates the transitory endocrine organ that secretes progesterone, known as the corpus luteum, whose main function is to prepare the endometrium, already proliferated by the action of follicular phase estrogens, for the implantation of the fertilized egg.

The endometrium expresses adhesion molecules that make it receptive to the blastocyst and between days 7 and 9 from ovulation, a period of maximum efficiency known as the window of implantation is established; after day 9, implantation is not possible, which is why it is called the refractory phase.

Eight or nine days after ovulation, at the time when implantation is expected, maximum vascularization is reached, the basal lamina dissolves, and the capillaries invade the granulosa cell layers in response to the secretion of angiogenic factors, both from the granulosa and from the theca cells, in harmony with the maximum levels of plasma progesterone and estradiol.

The survival of the corpus luteum depends on the continuous stimulation of LH, but estradiol metabolites, acting via paracrine-autocrine pathways, affect angiogenesis or LH-mediated events also [23].

The function of the corpus luteum decreases at the end of the luteal phase unless chorionic gonadotropin appears due to an eventual pregnancy. If pregnancy does not occur, the corpus luteum undergoes luteolysis. Under the action of estradiol and prostaglandins, it forms a scar tissue called *corpus albicans* [24].

As noted, estrogen levels increase and decrease twice during the menstrual cycle, increase during the middle follicular phase, and then decrease rapidly after ovulation, followed by a further increase during the middle luteal phase, in parallel with the increase in serum levels of progesterone and 17α-hydroxyprogesterone, all falling at the end of the menstrual cycle (**Figure 1**).

The mechanism of how the corpus luteum regulates steroid secretion is not known exactly. It may be determined in part by the pattern of LH secretion, changes in its receptor, or variations in the levels of enzymes that regulate the production of steroid hormones. The amount of granulosa cells formed during the follicular phase and the levels of LDL cholesterol that surround it may also play a role in the regulation of steroid synthesis by the corpus luteum.

There are at least two types of luteal cells, large and small.

Both produce progesterone but with differences. Large cells come from granulosa, are more active in steroidogenesis, produce large amounts of progesterone, and although they have numerous LH receptors, they do not elevate progesterone secretion in response to LH or cAMP. Instead, they possess receptors for PGF2a and respond to this hormone with activation of at least two second messengers. Activation of protein kinase C (PKC) decreases progesterone's secretion.

As a result of the binding of PGF2a to its receptor, the concentration of free intracellular calcium increases, which seems to be related to the induction of apoptosis and cell death.

The large cells are influenced by other autocrine and paracrine factors, such as inhibin, relaxin, and oxytocin (**Figure 16**). The small cells are derived from the theca, contain receptors for LH, and respond to LH or cAMP by increasing the secretion of progesterone by 5–15 times [25, 26].

The synthesis of progesterone by the corpus luteum is essential for the establishment and maintenance of pregnancy.

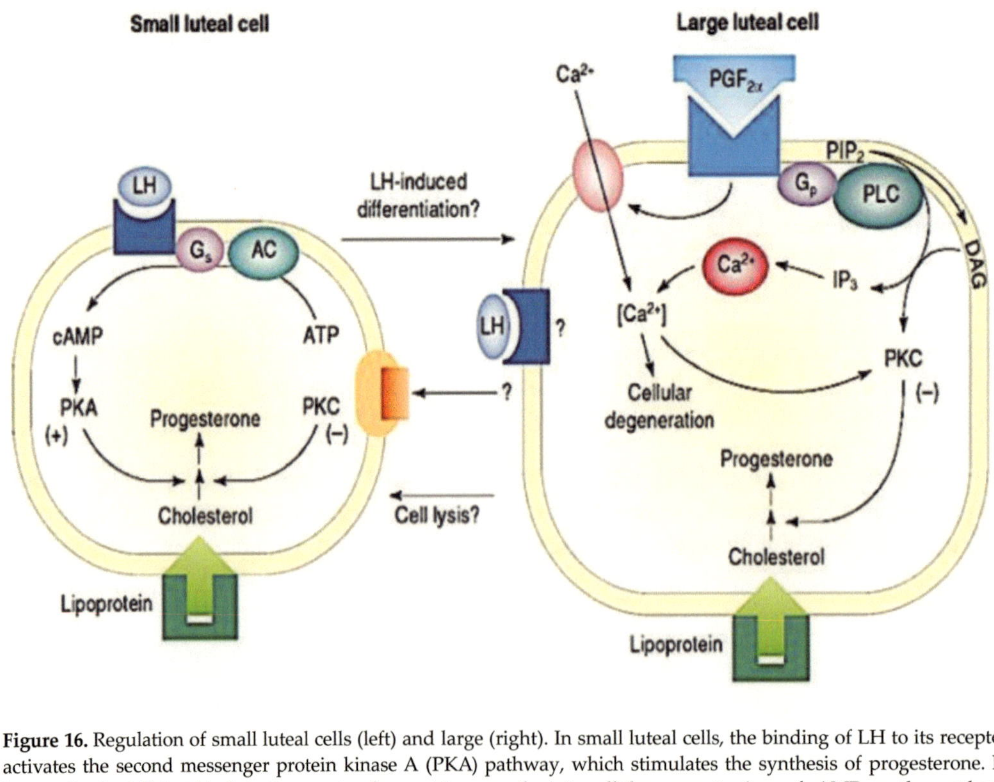


**Figure 16.** Regulation of small luteal cells (left) and large (right). In small luteal cells, the binding of LH to its receptor activates the second messenger protein kinase A (PKA) pathway, which stimulates the synthesis of progesterone. In large cells, the LH that binds to its receptor does not increase the intracellular concentrations of cAMP nor the synthesis of progesterone, but the binding of PGF2a to its receptor activates PKC, which inhibits the synthesis of progesterone and causes an influx of calcium that leads to cell degeneration. AC: adenylate cyclase, DAG: diacylglycerol, IP3: inositol 1,4,5-trisphosphate, PIP2: phosphatidylinositol 4,5-bisphosphate, and PLC: phospholipase C. From Niswender [25].

In addition to luteinization, that is, the conversion of an ovulatory follicle into the corpus luteum and luteal regression to allow a new cycle, there are also mechanisms of luteal maintenance and rescue to sustain pregnancy.

Humans preferably use circulating LDL cholesterol for steroidogenesis although the corpus luteum has the ability to synthesize its own cholesterol, in smaller amounts [27].

Inside the cells, lipid steroid precursors are found as free cholesterol. There is also esterified cholesterol that accumulates within the rough endoplasmic reticulum and as cytoplasmic lipid droplets or lipoprotein particles. These fatty acid esters of cholesterol cannot replace free cholesterol as a structural ingredient of the plasma membrane nor serve as direct substrates for the production of steroids. They are hydrolyzed by a neutral cholesterol ester hydrolase (NCEH), also known as hormone-sensitive lipase, because their activity is tightly regulated in steroidogenic tissues by FSH, LH, and hCG.

Progesterone secretion and estradiol during luteal phase is tightly connected with the pulses of secretion of LH (**Figure 12**). The frequency and widening of secretion of LH during follicular phase regulates the function of the posterior luteal phase and is concordant with the function of LH during luteal phase.

The frequency and widening of the pulses of secretion of pituitary LH affect the secretion of progesterone and estradiol during the luteal phase (**Figure 12**).

The half-life of the corpus luteum can be reduced with the continuous administration of LH during any of the phases, follicular or luteal, as if the LH concentration is lower or its pulses are reduced.

The luteal phase can suffer shortening also if the levels of FSH are inadequate or low, during the follicular phase, conditioning the development of a smaller corpus luteum.

The function of the corpus luteum begins to decrease 9–11 days after ovulation. The mechanism by which the corpus luteum undergoes involution (luteolysis) is partially elucidated. Prostaglandin F2α would have a luteolytic action, through the synthesis of endothelin-1 that inhibits steroidogenesis and stimulates the release of a growth factor, the tumor necrosis factor alpha (TNFα) oxytocin, and vasopressin and would produce a luteotropic effect through an autocrine/paracrine mechanism.

The ability of LH to negatively regulate its own receptor may also play a role at the end of the luteal phase; thereby, the involution of the corpus luteum must be caused by a decrease in the sensitivity of the LH receptors, rather than by a pulsatile secretion of it. Finally, the matrix metalloproteinases would also play a role in luteolysis and, therefore, in the fall of progesterone levels.

## 6. Menstruation

In the absence of pregnancy, the levels of progesterone and estradiol begin to decrease as a result of the corpus luteum decreasing. The fall of progesterone increases in degree of coiling and the constriction of the spiraled arterioles. This finally produces tissue ischemia due to decreased blood flow from the superficial, spongy, and compact endometrial layers. After the fall of serum concentrations of ovarian steroids, matrix metalloproteinases play a key role in the onset of menstrual bleeding in the human endometrium, by inducing the degradation of the extracellular matrix of this mucosa [28]. Endometrial prostaglandins cause contractions of the uterine smooth muscle and detachment of degraded tissue.

The release of prostaglandins may appear due to instability of the lysosomal membranes in the endometrial cells. The magnitude of this effect is such that inhibitors of prostaglandin synthesis can be used as a therapy in women with excessive uterine bleeding. Menstrual flow is composed of detachment of endometrial tissue, red blood cells, inflammatory exudates, and proteolytic enzymes.

Two days after the start of menstruation and while the shedding of the endometrium still occurs, the estrogen produced by the new growing follicles begins to stimulate the regeneration of the superficial layers of the endometrium. The estrogen secreted by the growing follicles causes a long constriction of the vessel facilitating the formation of a veil over the denuded endometrial vessels.

The average duration of menstruation is 4–6 days, but the normal range can be 2–8 days. As mentioned above, the average amount of bleeding loss is 30 ml and more than 80 ml is considered abnormal. A few years ago, a classification has been generalized to describe the abnormalities of bleeding suggested by the International Federation of Gynecology and Obstetrics [29].

### 6.1. Types of endometrium at echographies

The characteristics of the endometrium in gynecological ultrasound change depending on the period of the menstrual cycle, presenting different thicknesses according to the stage of the menstrual cycle (**Figure 17**).

**Endometrium type 0, postmenstrual:** it is characterized because only a fine refractive line can be seen. It is the endometrium typical of postmenopause, postpartum, or after a uterine scraping. Most postmenopausal women are between 3 and 5 mm thick, but it is normal up to 8 mm if there has been no unexpected bleeding.

**Endometrium type 1, preovulatory:** trilaminar endometrium, refers to the observation of three refractive lines. This stage corresponds to the proliferative or estrogenic phase. In an early follicular stage, the size of the endometrium is between 3 and 4 mm thick, while in the stage close to ovulation, it can reach 9–11 mm.

**Endometrium type 2, postovulatory:** in this stage, the progesterone matures the already proliferated endometrium, especially in its glandular and vascular structures, thickening the endometrium. The ultrasound image becomes whiter to the extent that it contains more water and glycogen. This layer of refringency represents most of the endometrium toward the end of the luteal phase.

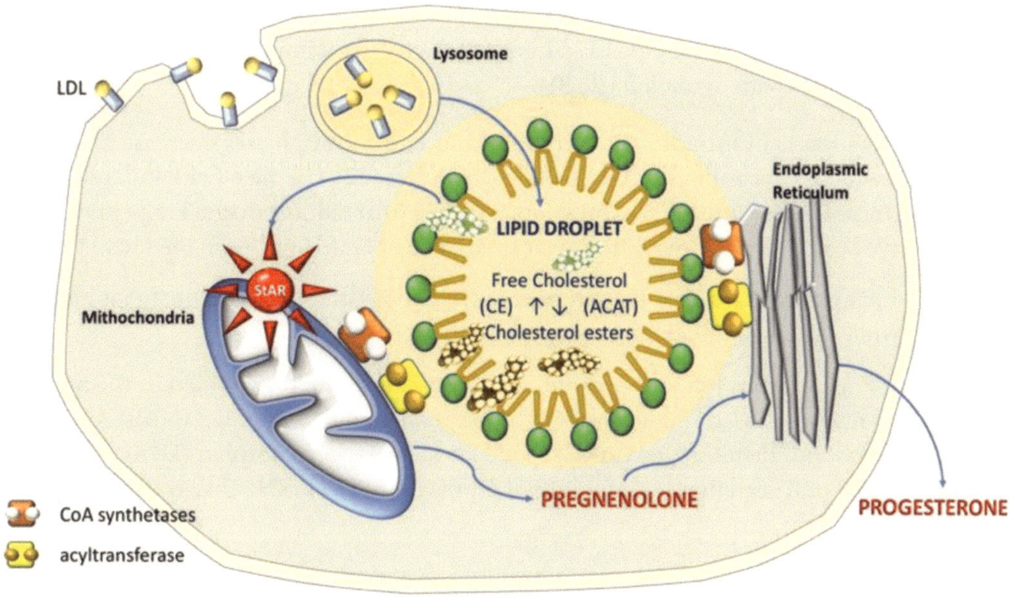


**Figure 17.** The main substrate for human steroidogenesis is LDL cholesterol: it is incorporated by endocytosis and stored as free cholesterol or as ester. Esterified cholesterol is hydrolyzed cholesterol esterases (CE) and transported as free cholesterol to the mitochondria. It passes from the outer mitochondrial membrane to the internal membrane, with the concurrence of the steroidogenic acute regulatory protein (StAR), peripheral type benzodiazepine receptors and endozepine. In mitochondria, cholesterol is converted to pregnenolone by cytochrome P450scc, which is transported out of the mitochondria and converted to progesterone by 3b-hydroxysteroid dehydrogenase, D5, D4 isomerase (3b-HSD), which is present in the smooth endoplasmic reticulum (The cell nucleus is not shown.)

**Endometrium type 3, premenstrual:** in this stage, there is only one large refractive line and corresponds to the late secretory phase.

### 6.2. Endocrine regulation of the menstrual cycle

When the gonadal axis has reached maturity, the neurons of the preoptic area and the infundibular and arcuate nuclei in the hypothalamus secrete GnRh in a pulsatile fashion, every 60–90 minutes, to the pituitary portal system.

Frequency and amplitude are essential to produce and maintain the effect on the gonadotropic cells of the anterior part of the pituitary gland, which consists of releasing both LH and FSH. The secreted amounts of each will depend not only on the pulsatility of GnRH, but also on the positive and negative feedbacks mechanisms of sex steroids.

In general, estrogen sensitizes and counter-regulates FSH, at both levels, the hypothalamus and the adenohypophysis, selectively modulated by other factors such as inhibins A and B. LH is sensitive to positive feedback, while there are estrogens in the late follicular phase and in the luteal phase, but the feedback becomes negative when estrogen levels fall at the end of the cycle.

Recent evidence indicates that the administration of progesterone in the late well-estrogenized follicular phase does not prevent the LH surge, which is of great importance because it would have no interference with ovulation [30, 31].

Relatively, low levels of estradiol, in early follicular and luteal phases, decrease kisspeptin expression, which reduces the amplitude of GnRH pulses [32]. On the other hand, progesterone would increase the dynorphin expression, which in turn reduces that of kisspeptin. These changes have been associated with the lower frequency of GnRH pulses in the luteal phase.

Other modulators that stimulate the pulsatile secretion of GnRH are glutamate and norepinephrine, while GABA and endogenous opioids inhibit it.

Neurokinin B and dynorphin neuropeptides act in an auto-synaptic fashion in the arcuate/infundibular nucleus, so that an increase in the expression of neurokinin B (NKB) stimulates the secretion of and, therefore, of GnRH, while an increase in dynorphin (Dyn) expression decreases kisspeptin secretion by inhibiting the pulsatility of GnRH. This system is known as KNDy [33].

At the beginning of the menstrual cycle, estradiol levels are low and FSH levels are slightly elevated. This ratio manages to recruit follicles and as that happens, not only estradiol increases but also inhibin A, due to the empowerment of FD, which generates a continuous decrease in FSH in the follicular phase.

The concentrations of FSH reach the maximum levels on the day when the FD is defined, followed by a slow decrease during the follicular phase, from day 5 to 13, reaching a nadir and then a peak just before ovulation (**Figure 14**). There comes a time when estradiol levels are such that they trigger the peak of FSH and LH, producing ovulation.

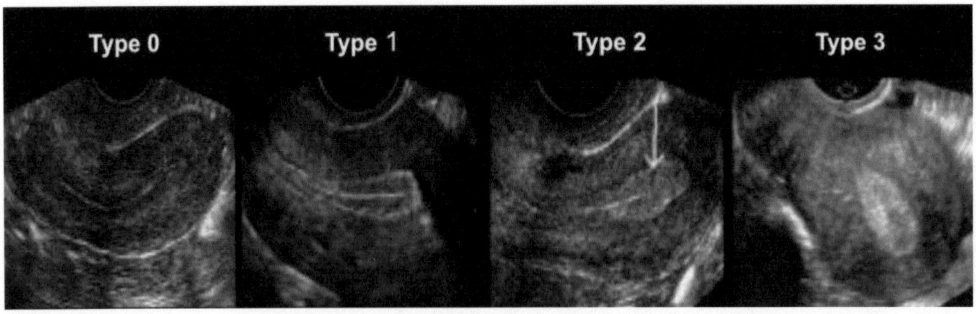


**Figure 18.** Types of endometrium in transvaginal ultrasound. The endometrium was classified into four types (0, 1, 2, and 3) according to the appearance of the myometrium-endometrium and endometrium-endometrium interfaces, the texture, and the thickness of the functional layer. Type 0: smooth, thin as a pencil line; type 1: trilaminar structure with an iso- or hypoechoic functional layer; type 2: also trilaminar, but the myometrium-endometrium interfaces are thicker than those of type 1; and type 3: thick and homogeneous echogenic image. The type of endometrium correlates with the day of the menstrual cycle. Ultrasound is defined on day 0 as the day of the follicle break. Type 0 is usually found on day −11, during and immediately after menstruation. Type 1 is observed during the middle follicular phase and until day +2. Types 2 and 3 are observed after the ovulatory days. The endometrium increases more thickness during the preovulatory phase (average +5.5 mm), and in the luteal phase, the average is +2.6 mm.

http://dx.doi.org/10.5772/intechopen.79876

As the luteal phase advance in time, inhibin A, estradiol, and progesterone fall together with the increase in activin A. FSH increases in the transition from the luteal phase to the next follicular phase, beginning 4 days before menstruation, a stage in which inhibin B increases during follicular recruitment.

The concentration of activin A secreted by the follicles increases in the second half of the luteal phase [34] (**Figure 18**), decreases at the beginning of the follicular phase, increases during the early follicular phase, and then increases during the middle follicular phase in parallel with estradiol and inhibin A (**Figure 19**).

In older women, FSH is higher, even during nadir, and the increase occurs early during the luteal phase. Recruitment of a group of follicles begins early, but the selection of DF is altered and can either advance or delay. The result is the variability of the cycle at the expense of a variable follicular phase, called "lag phase," which ends when the ETO is produced [35].

The ETO is when the estradiol overt elevation is achieved, which marks the selection of the FD. If an FD capable of ovulating was not achieved, the woman can go through a hyperestrogenic state without establishing a corpus luteum, so at the endometrial level, the cycle is hormonally monophasic. This is the pathophysiological basis that explains the monophasic hyperestrogenism that affects approximately one-third of women in perimenopause (**Figure 20**).

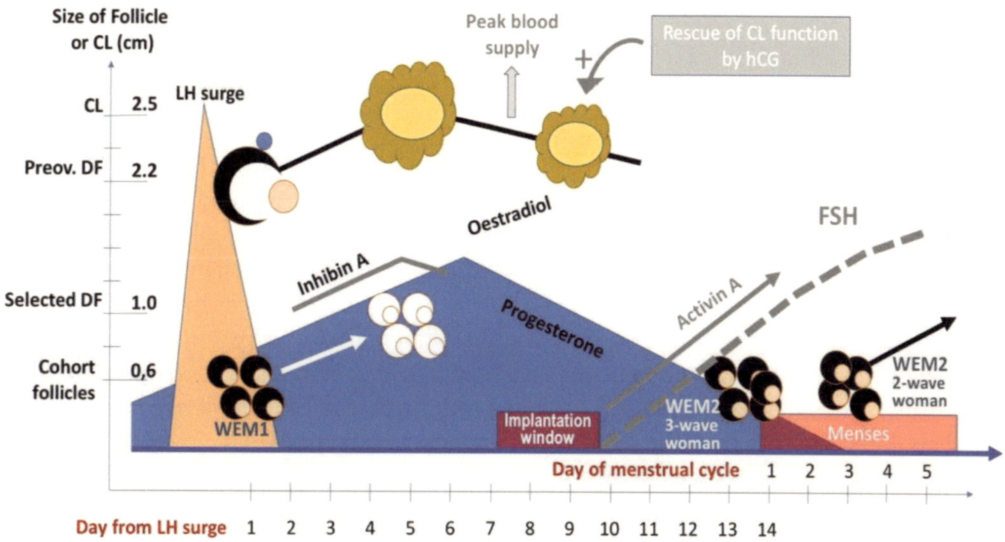


**Figure 19.** Scheme composed shows luteal events, follicular ones and hormonals during luteal phase of woman CL = corpus luteum; DF = dominant follicle; WEM1–3 = wave emergency 1, 2, or 3 at the cycle; the waves of follicle of light gray color indicates the low frequency of the principal waves (selection of DF) during luteal phase or early follicular ones in women of 2 or 3 waves. The estradiol rise in the follicular phase begins after the emergence of the ovulatory DF and becomes more rapid following DF selection, and occurs earlier in women with 2 versus 3 follicle waves per cycle. After ovulation, estradiol concentrations increase to the mid-luteal phase (days 7–9 after ovulation) and then decline, and this is due to luteal estradiol secretion and is unaffected by minor or major anovulatory waves. Adapted from Macklon and Fauser [5].

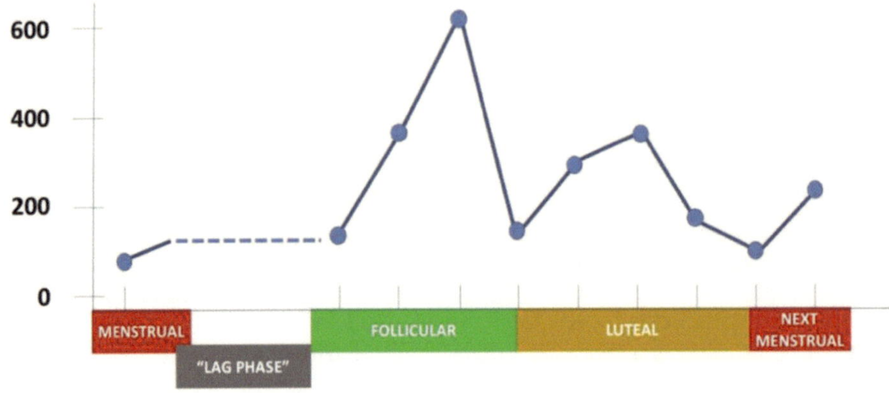


**Figure 20.** The variability in perimenopause depends on the lag phase, a delayed recruitment process. Adapted from Hale et al. [35].

A chronic negative energy imbalance reduces the pulsatility of LH, generates atresia of FD and, consequently, anovulation and amenorrhea. Weight loss is associated with a reduction in LH pulses, which generates functional, reversible hypothalamic amenorrhea. On the contrary, the pulsatility of LH is increased in adolescents with irregular cycles or in women with polycystic ovary syndrome, associated with anovulation also, but here the selection of DF is absent.

## 7. Conclusion

Human reproduction depends on the integrity of a system of intracrine and paracrine signals within the ovaries, in which those recruited follicles that have reached a level of differentiation that make them sensitive to the endocrine control of the other distant and great actor, the hypothalamus axis participate pituitary. Once a dominant follicle has been achieved, the elevations of the circulating levels of estradiol and inhibin B produced by it will modulate FSH levels and will allow, on the one hand, the atresia of the other follicles, and on the other, they will facilitate the LH surge, necessary to trigger ovulation. After hatching, the surrounding theca and granulosa cells from the follicular bed abandoned by the newly ovulated egg interact to produce a corpus luteum, which retains sufficient steroidogenic properties to produce progesterone at the concentration required to regulate the endometrium, till the implantation of a fertilized egg. If pregnancy does not occur, since the end of the luteal phase, gonadotropic changes are prepared to allow the development of a follicular recruitment phase.

Being such a complex process, dependent on so many variables and exposed to so many actions, reactions and interferences, the sequences of the menstrual cycle are remarkably predictable within not very wide ranges of variability. In general, the duration standards of each cycle, 25–35 days, coincide with the ovulation presumption criteria accepted for women with ovulatory anomalies such as in the polycystic ovarian syndrome. The detailed understanding of the mechanisms allow to improve the efficiency in the clinical management when it is intended to give assistance to obtain a pregnancy, as well as to avoid it when the goal is contraception, or to correct bleeding anomalies that may result from ovulatory disorders with luteal insufficiency. There are still many aspects to investigate.

## Conflict of interest

The authors declare no conflict of interest in relation to this publication.

## Author details

Barriga-Pooley Patricio[1]* and Brantes-Glavic Sergio[2]

*Address all correspondence to: pbarriga@uft.cl

1 Obstetrics and Gynaecology Department, School of Medicine, Finis Terrae and San Sebastian Universities, Santiago, Chile

2 Depto Ginecología y Obstericia, Universidad de Chile, Santiago, Chile

## References

[1] Reed BG, Carr BR. The normal menstrual cycle and the control of ovulation. In: De Groot LJ, Chrousos G, Dungan K, Feingold KR, Grossman A, Hershman JM, et al., editors. Endotext [Internet]. South Dartmouth (MA): MDText.com, Inc.; 2000 (ver 2018 Aug 5.)

[2] Welt CK, Pagan YL, Smith PC, Rado KB, Hall JE. Control of follicle-stimulating hormone by estradiol and the inhibins: Critical role of estradiol at the hypothalamus during the luteal-follicular transition. The Journal of Clinical Endocrinology and Metabolism. 2003 Apr;**88**(4):1766-1771. DOI: 10.1210/jc.2002-021516

[3] Mihm M, Gangooly S, Muttukrishna S. The normal menstrual cycle in women. Animal Reproduction Science. 2011;**124**(3-4):229-236. DOI: 10.1016/j.anireprosci.2010.08.030

[4] Hodgen GD. The dominant ovarian follicle. Fertility and Sterility. 1982;**38**:281-300

[5] Macklon NS, Fauser BC. Aspects of ovarian follicle development throughout life. Hormone Research. 1999;**52**(4):161-170. DOI: 10.1159/000023456

[6] Richards JS, Ren YA, Candelaria N, Adams JE, Rajkovic A. Ovarian follicular theca cell recruitment, differentiation, and impact on fertility: 2017 update. Endocrine Reviews. Feb 1 2018;**39**(1):1-20. DOI: 10.1210/er.2017-00164

[7] Baird DT, Fraser IS. Blood production and ovarian secretion rates of esuadiol-17β and estrone in women throughout the menstrual cycle. The Journal of Clinical Endocrinology and Metabolism. 1974;**38**:1009-1017

[8] Doshi SB, Agarwal A. The role of oxidative stress in menopause. Journal of Midlife Health. 2013;**4**(3):140-146. DOI: 10.4103/0976-7800.118990

[9] Groome NP, Illingworth PJ, O'Brien M, Pai R, Rodger FE, Mather JP, et al. Measurement of dimeric inhibin B throughout the human menstrual cycle. The Journal of Clinical Endocrinology and Metabolism. 1996;**81**(4):1401-1405. DOI: 10.1210/jcem.81.4.8636341

[10] Welt CK, Martin KA, Taylor AE, Lambert-Messerlian GM, Crowley WF Jr, Smith JA, et al. Frequency modulation of follicle-stimulating hormone (FSH) during the luteal-follicular transition: Evidence for FSH control of inhibin B in normal women. The Journal of Clinical Endocrinology and Metabolism 1997;**82**(8):2645-2652. DOI: 10.1210/jcem.82.8.4138

[11] Small CM, Manatunga AK, Klein M, Feigelson HS, Dominguez CE, McChesney R, et al. Menstrual cycle characteristics: Associations with fertility and spontaneous abortion. Epidemiology. 2006 Jan;**17**(1):52-60

[12] Wilcox AJ, Dunson D, Baird DD. The timing of the "fertile window" in the menstrual cycle: Day specific estimates from a prospective study. BMJ. 2000;**321**(7271):1259-1262. DOI: 10.1136/bmj.321.7271.1259

[13] Wise LA, Mikkelsen EM, Rothman KJ, Riis AH, Sørensen HT, Huybrechts KF, et al. A prospective cohort study of menstrual characteristics and time to pregnancy. American Journal of Epidemiology. 2011;**174**(6):701-709. DOI: 10.1093/aje/kwr130

[14] La Marca A, Broekmans FJ, Volpe A, Fauser BC, Macklon NS, ESHRE Special Interest Group for Reproductive Endocrinology–AMH Round Table. Anti-Mullerian hormone (AMH): What do we still need to know? Human Reproduction. 2009 Sep;**24**(9):2264-2275. DOI: 10.1093/humrep/dep210

[15] Broekmans FJ, Visser JA, Laven JS, Broer SL, Themmen AP, Fauser BC. Anti-Müllerian hormone and ovarian dysfunction. Trends in Endocrinology and Metabolism. 2008 Nov;**19**(9):340-347. DOI: 10.1016/j.tem.2008.08.002

[16] Sollenberger MJ, Carlsen EC, Johnson ML, Veldhuis JD, Evans WS. Specific physiological regulation of luteinizing hormone secretory events throughout the human menstrual cycle: New insights into the pulsatile mode of gonadotropin release. Journal of Neuroendocrinology. 1990;**2**(6):845-852. DOI: 10.1111/j.1365-2826.1990.tb00650.x

[17] Hoff JD, Quigley ME, Yen SCC. Hormonal dynamics at midcycle: A re-evaluation. The Journal of Clinical Endocrinology and Metabolism. 1983;**57**:792

[18] Irianni F, Hodgen GD. Mechanism of ovulation. Endocrinology and Metabolism Clinics of North America. 1992;**21**(1):19-38. DOI: 10.1016/S0889-8529(18)30230-5

[19] Jesam C, Salvatierra AM, Schwartz JL, Croxatto HB. Suppression of follicular rupture with meloxicam, a cyclooxygenase-2 inhibitor: Potential for emergency contraception. Human Reproduction. 2010;**25**(2):368-373. DOI: 10.1093/humrep/dep392

[20] Duffy DM. Novel contraceptive targets to inhibit ovulation: The prostaglandin E2 pathway. Human Reproduction Update. 2015;**21**(5):652-670. DOI: 10.1093/humupd/dmv026

[21] Russell DL, Robker RL. Molecular mechanisms of ovulation: Co-ordination through the cumulus complex. Human Reproduction Update. 2007;**13**(3):289-312. DOI: 10.1093/humupd/dml062

[22] Richards JS, Russell DL, Robker RL, Dajee M, Alliston TN. Molecular mechanisms of ovulation and luteinization. Molecular and Cellular Endocrinology. 1998;**145**(1-2):47-54. DOI: 10.1016/S0303-7207(98)00168-3

[23] Devoto L, Henríquez S, Kohen P, Strauss JF 3rd. The significance of estradiol metabolites in human corpus luteum physiology. Steroids. 2017;**123**:50-54. DOI: 10.1016/j.steroids.2017.05.002

[24] Stocco C, Telleria C, Gibori G. The molecular control of corpus luteum formation, function, and regression. Endocrine Reviews. 2007;**28**(1):117-149. DOI: 10.1210/er.2006-0022

[25] Niswender GD. Molecular control of luteal secretion of progesterone. Reproduction. 2002;**123**(3):333-339

[26] Niswender GD, Juengel JL, Silva PJ, Rollyson MK, McIntush EW. Mechanisms controlling the function and life span of the corpus luteum. Physiological Reviews. 2000;**80**(1):1-29. DOI: 10.1152/physrev.2000.80.1.1

[27] Christenson LK, Devoto L. Cholesterol transport and steroidogenesis by the corpus luteum. Reproductive Biology and Endocrinology. 2003;**1**:90. DOI: 10.1186/1477-7827-1-90

[28] Henriet P, Cornet PB, Lemoine P, Galant C, Singer CF, Courtoy PJ, et al. Circulating ovarian steroids and endometrial matrix metalloproteinases (MMPs). Annals of the New York Academy of Sciences. 2002;**955**:119-138. DOI: 10.1111/j.1749-6632.2002.tb02773.x

[29] Munro MG, Critchley HO, Broder MS, Fraser IS, FIGO Working Group on Menstrual Disorders. FIGO classification system (PALM-COEIN) for causes of abnormal uterine bleeding in nongravid women of reproductive age. International Journal of Gynaecology and Obstetrics. 2011;**113**(1):3-13. DOI: 10.1016/j.ijgo.2010.11.011

[30] Hutchens EG, Ramsey KA, Howard LC, Abshire MY, Patrie JT, McCartney CR. Progesterone has rapid positive feedback actions on LH release but fails to reduce LH pulse frequency within 12 h in estradiol-pretreated women. Physiological Reports. 2016;**4**(16). DOI: 10.14814/phy2.12891

[31] Kim SH, Burt Solorzano CM, McCartney CR. Progesterone administration does not acutely alter LH pulse secretion in the mid-follicular phase in women. Physiological Reports. 2018;**6**(8):e13680. DOI: 10.14814/phy2.13680

[32] Skorupskaite K, George JT, Anderson RA. The kisspeptin-GnRH pathway in human reproductive health and disease. Human Reproduction Update. 2014;**20**(4):485-500. DOI: 10.1093/humupd/dmu009

[33] Lehman MN, Coolen LM, Goodman RL. Minireview: Kisspeptin/neurokinin B/dynorphin (KNDy) cells of the arcuate nucleus: A central node in the control of gonadotropin-releasing hormone secretion. Endocrinology. 2010;**151**(8):3479-3489. DOI: 10.1210/en.2010-0022

[34] Bilezikjian LM, Blount AL, Leal AM, Donaldson CJ, Fischer WH, Vale WW. Autocrine/paracrine regulation of pituitary function by activin, inhibin and follistatin. Molecular and Cellular Endocrinology. 2004 Oct 15;**225**(1-2):29-36. DOI: 10.1016/j.mce.2004.02.010

[35] Hale GE, Zhao X, Hughes CL, Burger HG, Robertson DM, Fraser IS. Endocrine features of menstrual cycles in middle and late reproductive age and the menopausal transition classified according to the staging of reproductive aging workshop (STRAW) staging system. The Journal of Clinical Endocrinology and Metabolism. 2007;**92**(8):3060-3067

Chapter 3

# Pre Menstrual Syndrome

Preye Fiebai, Avwebo Ochuko Ukueku and
Rosemary Ogu

Additional information is available at the end of the chapter

http://dx.doi.org/10.5772/intechopen.80492

**Abstract**

Approximately 80–90% of women experience some symptoms in the premenstrual period at some point in their reproductive years. Teenagers often present with moderate to severe symptoms, while women in the fourth decade of life appear to have worse symptoms with the severity of the disease worsening with increasing age up until menopause. Obesity and smoking have also been identified as risk factors. Symptoms could be physical, psychological, emotional, environmental and/or behavioral and affect the ability to perform normal daily activities as well as adversely affect interpersonal relationships. Though several theories have been propounded, the exact cause of premenstrual syndrome is unknown. Management of this disorder requires a multi-disciplinary approach involving the general practitioner, the general gynecologist or a gynecologist with a special interest in PMS, a mental health professional (psychiatrist, clinical psychologist or counselor), physiotherapist and dietician.

**Keywords:** menstruation, psychosomatic menstrual syndrome, girls

## 1. Introduction

A syndrome is a group of symptoms and/or signs associated with a medical disease or disorder, often occurring concurrently. Premenstrual syndrome (PMS) can be defined as a group of physical and emotional symptoms and signs usually occurring within the last 14 days of the menstrual cycle, that is, from ovulation to the onset of menstruation, of sufficient severity to result in deterioration of interpersonal relationships and affect normal activities [1]. The symptoms span a range of medical specialties; from the gynecological to the psychiatric. PMS is included as a diagnostic category in the 10th edition of the International Statistical Classification of Diseases and Related Health Problems (ICD) with its' more "severe" form,

Premenstrual Dysphoric Disorder (PMDD), included in the 5th edition of the Diagnostic and Statistical Manual for Mental Disorders (DSM) [1, 2].

Premenstrual syndrome became a recognized medical disorder over the last century. It was initially thought to be an 'imagined' disease all in the heads of 'crazy' women [3]. Later it was presumed that the female reproductive organs had complete control over the woman and energies diverted from reproductive organs caused suboptimal functioning as such women involved in manual labor required more treatments than those who only exercised their brains [4]. Till date, symptoms of PMS are often viewed with skepticism or used in mockery of the female sex or the idealism of gender equality such that many females who suffer from this condition are unwilling to seek help or even admit to having difficulty managing the psychological symptoms associated with their menstrual cycles. This chapter methodology derives from a synthesis of the available literature under the MESH search term premenstrual and focus group discussion of women attending a tertiary health facility in Southern Nigeria.

Premenstrual syndrome was named by a British physician Katharina Dalton in 1953 [5]. PMS psychological symptoms had been described as early as the time of the ancient Greeks, but it wasn't until 1931 that this disorder was recognized by the medical community. This diagnosis was made popular by a paper presented at the New York Academy of Medicine by Robert T. Frank titled "Hormonal Causes of Premenstrual Tension" [6]. Robert Frank theorized that excess estrogen levels were the cause of symptoms experienced by affected women. In 1981, Dalton served as the chief defense medical expert in a murder trial in London. She successfully argued that the defendant was not responsible for murdering her lover because she suffered from severe PMS. This trial caught the attention of different viewers in the United States and brought publicity to PMS. PMS or the "disease of the 1980s" became a media event. More importantly, PMS acquired medical legitimacy, "after years of telling women their problems were 'all in the head,' the proportion of doctors who accepted PMS as a real disease reached critical mass" [7].

## 2. Epidemiology

Approximately 80–90% of women experience some symptoms in the premenstrual period at some point in their reproductive years. However, only 20% of these women meet the diagnostic criteria for PMS, of these; 10% are severely affected and 3–8% have PMDD [1].

Teenagers often present with moderate to severe symptoms, 14–88% of teenage girls are affected, with the older teenagers more likely to have symptoms than the younger teenagers. PMS and PMDD are associated with a higher risk of Anorexia nervosa, Bulimia nervosa and substance abuse. It is also more likely to occur in women who have suffered some form of abuse (emotional, physical or sexual) in early life or are presently in abusive relationships [8, 9].

Women in the fourth decade of life appear to have worse symptoms, and the severity of the disease tends to worsen with increasing age up until menopause. There is also an increased risk of hypertensive disorders in affected patients later in life.

http://dx.doi.org/10.5772/intechopen.80492

There is evidence of genetic predisposition to the disease as women whose mothers suffered from PMS are at higher risk of having the disease, and also monozygotic twins have a 93% rate of PMS compared with 44% in dizygotic twins [9]. Symptoms also vary with race; while black women often experience a higher prevalence of food cravings than white women, the white women often experience a higher prevalence of mood swings and weight gain [10].

Obesity and smoking have also been identified as risk factors for this condition. Women with body mass index more than 30, are three times more likely to have PMS than non-obese women and women who smoke are more than two times likely to present with severe symptoms [10, 11].

## 3. Clinical presentation

PMS symptoms tend to occur in a cyclic pattern from ovulation to onset of menstruation. Symptoms could be physical, psychological/emotional, environmental and/or behavioral [12, 13]. Over 200 symptoms have been described. Symptoms and signs tend to affect a patient's ability to perform normal daily activities and adversely affect their interpersonal relationships. Occasionally it results in violence in the home and broken marriages as well as loss of a woman's economic means in society. In a focus group discussion carried out among women attending a tertiary health facility in Southern Nigeria, premenstrual syndrome was viewed as a curse because of its myriad of symptoms.

Physical symptoms include the following:

Headaches

Acne

Breast tenderness

Abdominal bloating

Diarrhea or constipation

Joint and muscle pains

Fatigue

Weight gain (from fluid retention)

Swelling of the extremities

Dysmenorrhea

Change in bowel habits

Frequent urination

Hot flashes or cold sweats

General aches or pains (malaise)

Nausea and vomiting

Allergic reactions

Upper respiratory tract infections

Palpitations

Unusual food cravings

Low tolerance for noise, odors or light

Psychological/emotional symptoms include the following:

- Anxiety symptoms such as:

  Difficulty sleeping

  Tense feelings

  Irritability

  Clumsiness

  Mood swings

  Panic attacks

  Paranoia

- Depressive symptoms such as:

  Depressed mood and affect

  Angry feelings for no reason

  Feelings that are easily upset

  Poor concentration

  Memory loss

  Feelings of low self-worth

  Violent feelings and/or action

  Crying spells

  Social withdrawal

  Changes in appetite

  Changes in libido

Mental health disorders are worsened or exacerbated by PMS. These include depression and anxiety disorders. Other medical conditions whose symptoms may be worsened by PMS include; myalgic encephalomyelitis or chronic fatigue syndrome, irritable bowel syndrome and bladder pain syndrome. Health problems such as asthma, allergies and migraines may also worsen with this disease. Patients with PMS may also experience heavy menstrual bleeding and early menopause.

## 4. The pathophysiology of premenstrual syndrome

The exact cause of premenstrual syndrome is unknown and is the subject of much ongoing research. Several theories have been proposed; from sex hormones interactions to neurotransmitters interactions in the central nervous system. Older theories that have proven to be incorrect include estrogen excess or withdrawal, progesterone deficiency (these were the initial sex hormones theories), pyridoxine (vitamin B6) deficiency, alteration of glucose metabolism, fluid-electrolyte imbalances. Current research provides some evidence supporting the following etiologies:

### 4.1. Sex hormone

Symptoms of premenstrual syndrome begin following ovulation and resolve with menses, and because they only affect women in reproductive age, it is assumed that the female gonadal hormones (estrogen and progestogen) have a role in the pathophysiology of the disease. This is underscored by the facts that symptoms are less common in women with surgical oophorectomy or drug-induced ovarian hypofunction, such as with gonadotropin-releasing hormone (GnRH) agonists. Moreover, women with anovulatory cycles rarely report PMS symptoms. For these reasons, research of PMS pathophysiology has focused on the sex steroids, estrogen and progesterone. However, no propounded theory so far has borne fruit.

### 4.2. Serotonin deficiency

It is postulated that patients with PMS suffer from lower serotonin level in the luteal phase, which may or may not be as a result of the various interactions of the sex hormones. It has been proven that patients most affected by symptoms of PMS have differences in serotonin levels when compare to others. This evidence supports a role for serotonergic system dysregulation in the pathophysiology of PMS. Moreover, trials of serotonergic treatments have shown symptom reduction in women with PMS, symptoms respond to selective serotonin reuptake inhibitors (SSRIs), which increase the levels of circulating serotonin.

### 4.3. Central nervous system interaction

Estrogen and progesterone are neuroactive steroids and influence the central nervous system (CNS) neurotransmitters: serotonin, noradrenaline, and γ-aminobutyric acid (GABA). The predominant action of estrogen is neuronal excitability, whereas progestogens are inhibitory. Women with PMS have exaggerated responses to normal levels of these hormones, and rapid changes in the levels of these hormones as is experienced in the luteal phase of the menstrual cycle promote the development of symptoms.

### 4.4. Nutrient deficiencies

Magnesium and calcium deficiencies have been hypothesized to be causes of PMS symptoms. Studies evaluating supplemental therapies have shown improvement in symptoms.

### 4.5. Psychosocial theory

The psychosocial theory postulates that PMS is a conscious demonstration of a woman's conflict with her femininity and motherhood. It suggests that the premenstrual physical changes remind the woman that she is not fulfilling her traditional role of incubating, nurturing, and rearing a child. This theory is highly subjective and scientifically unprovable.

### 4.6. Sociocultural theory

The sociocultural theory postulates that PMS is a manifestation of a conflict between the societal expectation of the dual role of a woman as both a productive part of the workforce and a mother. It suggests that PMS is a cultural expression of women's dissatisfaction with their traditional roles in society.

### 4.7. Cognitive and social learning theory

This theory suggests that the onset of menstrual bleeding is an adverse psychological outcome for some women and PMS is a display of maladaptive coping strategies in other to reduce immediate stress.

## 5. Diagnosis of premenstrual syndrome

Diagnosis of PMS can often be difficult because may medical and psychological conditions mimic the symptoms, and there are no laboratory tests to confirm the diagnosis. Women with PMS usually present with complaints from multiple systems, and these symptoms display temporal association with the menstrual cycle luteal phase. Symptoms must begin at least 5 days (American College of Obstetricians and Gynecologists [ACOG] criteria) [8] or 1 week (DSM-IV-TR) before menses, and remit within 4 days (ACOG criteria) or a few days (DSM-IV-TR) after menses onset [2]. Evaluation of women complaining of PMS symptoms includes prospective daily symptom rating for at least two or three menstrual cycles.

A menstrual diary could be used to record the onset and duration of symptoms of PMS for 2–3 cycles; this not only helps the physician make the diagnosis but also increases the patient's awareness of her body and moods. She is thus, better at coping with her symptoms. The Endicott Daily Record of Problem Severity chart or the Daily Symptom Rating are tools that can be used to assess the frequency and severity of symptoms described in the luteal phase as against those experienced in the follicular phase of the menstrual cycle [14].

A within-cycle increase from follicular to luteal phase score of at least 20–50% is necessary to confirm a diagnosis of PMS. This is calculated by subtracting the follicular score from the luteal score, divided by the luteal score and multiplied by 100 (luteal score – follicular score/luteal score × 100).

A physical examination may identify some of the physical symptoms and signs of the disease. In certain instances, PMS symptoms may be an exacerbation of underlying primary psychiatric condition(s). Thus, a psychiatric evaluation may help rule out other common psychiatric conditions such as depression, dysthymia, and anxiety disorders. Additionally, other medical conditions that have a multisystem presentation should be considered. These include hypothyroidism, systemic lupus erythematosus, endometriosis, anemia, fibromyalgia, chronic fatigue syndrome, fibrocystic breast disease, irritable bowel syndrome, and migraine. Laboratory studies should include complete blood count, thyroid function tests and gynecological hormone profile.

## 6. Premenstrual dystrophic disorder (PMDD)

This is a condition in which a woman has severe depressive symptoms, tension and irritability before menstruation. It is a more severe form of PMS that affects a small percentage of women within reproductive age resulting in remarkable disability and loss of function. Symptoms are of sufficient severity as to interfere with work or school, social activities, interpersonal relationships and quality of life. Patients complain of similar symptoms as seen in PMS but of increased severity. Most symptoms of PMDD are similar to symptoms of a major depressive disorder (MDD). These symptoms, however, are cyclic and disappear with the onset of menses. The most common symptoms of PDMM are irritability, limited concentration, sleep disturbance, mood lability and marked depressed mood. Similarities to MDD are highlighted below.

- Markedly depressed mood. A symptom of MDD is depressed mood most of the day, nearly every day.
- Decreased interest in usual activities. One criterion for MDD is markedly diminished interest or pleasure in all activities.
- Lethargy, fatigability or lack of energy. Similarly, patients with MDD have fatigue or loss of energy.
- Hypersomnia or insomnia—also symptoms of MDD.

## 7. Diagnosis

The Diagnostic and Statistical Manual of Mental Disorders, 5th edition established 7 criteria for diagnosis of PMDD [2] (A–G).

### 7.1. Criterion A

In Criterion A in most menstrual cycles during the past year, 5 out of 11 symptoms listed must be present (including one of the first four) in the last 1–2 weeks before the onset of menses and disappear in the week post-menses. These symptoms are as follows:

1. Marked lability (mood swings)
2. Marked irritability or anger
3. Marked depressed mood
4. Marked anxiety or tension
5. Decreased interest in usual activities
6. Difficulty in concentration
7. Lethargy and marked lack of energy
8. Marked change in appetite (overeating or special food cravings)
9. Hypersomnia or insomnia
10. Feeling overwhelmed or out of control
11. Physical symptoms (e.g. breast tenderness, bloating, weight gain or swelling of extremities etc.)

### 7.2. Criterion B

One of the following symptoms must be present:

1. Marked affective lability
2. Marked irritability or anger or increased interpersonal conflicts
3. Marked depressed mood, feelings of hopelessness or self-deprecating thoughts
4. Marked anxiety tension and/or feelings of being keyed up or on edge.

### 7.3. Criterion C

One or more of the following symptoms must be present additionally, to reach a total of five symptoms when combined with Criterion B.

1. Decreased interest in usual activities (e.g. work, school, hobbies, friends)
2. Subjective difficulty in concentrating
3. Lethargy, easy fatigability, or marked lack of energy
4. Marked change in appetite (overeating or specific food cravings)
5. Hypersomnia or insomnia

6. Feeling overwhelmed or out of control
7. Physical symptoms (e.g. breast tenderness, bloating, weight gain or swelling of extremities)

Note: the symptoms in criteria A–C must be met for most of the menstrual cycles in the preceding year.

### 7.4. Criterion D

The symptoms are associated with clinically significant distress or interference with work, school, usual social activities or relationship with others (e.g. avoidance of social activities, decreased productivity and efficiency at work, school, or home).

### 7.5. Criterion E

The disturbance is not merely an exacerbation of the symptoms of another disorder, such as a major depressive disorder, panic disorder, persistent depressive disorder (dysthymia) or a personality disorder (although it may occur concurrently with any of these disorders).

### 7.6. Criterion F

Prospective daily ratings during at least two symptomatic cycles should confirm Criterion A. (Note: the diagnosis may be made provisionally prior to this confirmation).

### 7.7. Criterion G

The symptoms are not attributable to the physiological effects of a substance, (e.g. substance abuse, a medication, or other treatment) or another medical disorder (e.g. hyperthyroidism).

## 8. Management

### 8.1. Patient education/counseling

PMS may cause significant distress for patients especially the adolescents and as such providing patients with adequate information on the disease including alternative therapies is imperative. Management of this disorder requires a multi-disciplinary approach involving the general practitioner, the general gynecologist or a gynecologist with particular interest in PMS, a mental health professional (psychiatrist, clinical psychologist or counselor), physiotherapist and dietician.

### 8.2. Life style and dietary changes

Treatment of PMS is majorly according to the severity of symptoms [8, 12, 13, 15]. Regular exercise and dietary restrictions often reduce symptoms. Obese patients should be encouraged to join a weight management program. Dietary modification is often a part of the overall treatment regime. Patients are encouraged to consume smaller meal portions high in carbohydrates. Patients should be counseled to avoid salt, caffeine, alcohol and simple or refined sugars. Exercise and physical activities cause a release of endorphins which improve general health, nervous tension and anxiety.

### 8.3. Behavioral anger and stress management therapies

This may help patients cope and or regain control during times of heightened emotions. A variety of methods may be employed. These include; emotional support from family and friends, individual and couples' therapy, self-help support groups, anger management courses, stress management classes, as well as cognitive-behavioral therapy. Our clients described emotional support from family and friends as very helpful. Relaxation techniques such as yoga, biofeedback and self-hypnosis are also be helpful.

### 8.4. Supplements

These include but are not limited to calcium and magnesium supplements, vitamin E and B6, and polyunsaturated fatty acids (omega-3 and omega-6). Some alternative medicines/herbal supplements have been used to ease PMS symptoms with varying reports of success. These include; Black cohosh, Chaste berry (or vitex agnus-castus), Evening Primrose oil, St John's Wort and Dandelion. Research has shown that for these remedies to be effective, they need to be taken for at least two consecutive cycles. However, some of these remedies may be toxic and cause liver damage at high doses.

### 8.5. Medications

Various medications have been used to address the moderate to severe symptoms of PMS including:

*Diuretics*: These are often given to eliminate excess fluid. For example, spironolactone is widely used to treat swelling of the hands, feet and face.

*Hormonal therapies*: Some women benefit from combined oral contraceptives. The newer formulations (drospirenone-containing COCPs) control the fluctuations of the sex hormones reducing symptoms of PMS. The Mirena Intrauterine System releases low doses of progesterone and suppresses ovulation reducing the symptoms of PMS; however, it may initially induce PMS-like symptoms. Depo-Provera has a similar mechanism of action. Percutaneous estradiol combined with cyclical progestogens has been found to be useful in managing both physical and psychological symptoms of PMS.

*Gonadotrophin-releasing hormone (GnRH) analogues and agonists*: These are ovarian hormone suppressors, by suppressing the release of the sex hormones from the ovaries, they reduce the symptoms of PMS. GnRH analogues are highly effective in treating symptoms of severe PMS. An example of a GnRH analogue is danazol, and a GnRH agonist is goserelin. However, use of these therapies for greater than 6 months is associated with increased risk of osteoporosis and irreversible virilizing effects; therefore, in women receiving GnRH analogues for more than 6 months, add-back hormone therapy should be given. COCPs should be given or tibolone is recommended.

*Analgesics and anti-prostaglandins*: These are commonly used to treat menstrual cramps, headaches, breast tenderness and pelvic discomfort. Non-steroidal anti-inflammatory drugs like ibuprofen, naproxen and mefenamic acid have been very useful. However, long-term use may predispose patient to gastric ulcers.

*Antidepressants*: These increase levels of neurotransmitters and excitatory chemical in the brain (e.g. serotonin, GABA, opioids). They help treat mood disturbances associated with PMS. Examples include; fluoxetine and paroxetine.

*Selective serotonin reuptake inhibitors (SSRIs) and selective noradrenaline reuptake inhibitors (SNRIs)*: These are mood stabilizers with antidepressant effects. There increase the levels of serotonin and noradrenaline in the brain, both of which tend to decrease in the luteal phase in women with PMS.

### 8.6. Bilateral oophorectomy

In extreme cases, especially when the patient's quality of life is affected as seen in PMDD, and knowing the disease worsen with age, patients may be counseled for a bilateral oophorectomy and hysterectomy. This is especially recommended for patients who have completed their reproductive careers or patients who have severe symptoms unresponsive to all other therapies. It, however, tilts the women into early menopause with its problems as such hormone replacement therapies (HRT) should be considered. Bilateral oophorectomy without removal of the uterus will necessitate the use of a progestogen as part of HRT which carries the risk of PMS-like symptoms.

## 9. Conclusion

Premenstrual syndrome is a disease very prominent among women of reproductive age. It is not to be dismissed, taken for granted or treated with skepticism. There are therapies to end the sufferings of affected women. It is essential that we treat these women in other to promote their health, the health of the family and to sustain the economic productivity of women in our communities.

## Author details

Preye Fiebai[1,2], Avwebo Ochuko Ukueku[2] and Rosemary Ogu[1,2]*

*Address all correspondence to: rosemary.ogu@uniport.edu.ng

1 University of Port Harcourt, Port Harcourt, Nigeria

2 University of Port Harcourt Teaching Hospital, Port Harcourt, Nigeria

## References


[1] O'Brien S, Rapkin A, Dennerstein L, Nevatte T. Diagnosis and management of premenstrual disorders. BMJ. 2011;**342**:d2994

[2] American Psychiatric Association. Diagnostic and Statistical Manual of Mental Disorders (DSM-V). 5th ed. Washington, DC: APA; 2013

[3] Lane D. The curse of PMS. In: Evening Echo. Thomas Crosbie Holdings; July 2011. p. 11

[4] Martins E. Premenstrual syndrome, work, discipline and anger. In: Holmstrom N, editor. The Socialist Feminist Project: A Contemporary Reader in Theory and Politics. New York (USA): NYU Press; 2002. pp. 63-72

[5] Greene R, Dalton K. The premenstrual syndrome. BMJ. 1953;**1**:1007-1014

[6] Frank RT. The hormonal causes of premenstrual tension. Arch Neurol Psychiatry. Nov 1 1931;**26**(5):1053-1057

[7] Figert AE. Is PMS real? PMS as a scientific and cultural artifact. In: Women and the Ownership of PMS: The Structuring of a Psychiatric Disorder. 2nd ed. New Brunswick, USA: Transaction Publishers; 2007. pp. 6-7

[8] American College of Obstetricians and Gynecologists, ACOG. Premenstrual Syndrome (PMS). Washington, DC: ACOG; 2015. Available from: https://www.acog.org/Patients/FAQs/Premenstrual-Syndrome-PMS [cited 7/25/18]

[9] Dickerson LM, Mazyck PJ, Hunter MH. Premenstrual syndrome. American Family Physician. Apr 2003;**67**(8):1743-1752

[10] Bradshaw KD. Chapter 13. Psychosocial issues and female sexuality. In: Schorge JO, Schaffer JI, Halvorson LM, Hoffman BL, Bradshaw KD, Cunningham FG, editors. Williams Gynecology. 3rd ed. China: McGraw-Hill Companies Inc; 2008. pp. 625-629

[11] Khajehei M. Aetiology, diagnosis and management of premenstrual syndrome. Journal of Pain Relief. 2015;**4**:193

[12] Steiner M, Pearlstein T, Cohen LS. Expert Guidelines for the treatment of severe PMS, PMDD and comorbidities: The role of SSRIs. Journal of Women's Health (Larchmt). 2006;**15**(1):57-69

[13] Green LJ, O'Brien PMS, Panay N, Craig M, on behalf of the Royal College of Obstetricians and Gynaecologists. Management of premenstrual syndrome. Green-top guideline No. 48 February 2017. BJOG. 2017;**124**:e73-e105

[14] Endicott J, Nee J, Harrison W. Daily record of severity of problems (DRSP): Reliability and validity. Arch Womens Ment Health. Jan 2006;**9**(1):41-49

[15] Rapkin AJ, Lewis EI. Treatment of premenstrual dystrophic disorder. Women's Health. 2013;**9**(6):537-556

Chapter 4

# Secretory Phase and Implantation

Courtney Marsh, Katelyn Schumacher,
Warren B. Nothnick, Robert N. Taylor and
Monique Monard

Additional information is available at the end of the chapter

http://dx.doi.org/10.5772/intechopen.81304

**Abstract**

This chapter will explore the latter phase of the menstrual cycle focusing on the secretory phase of the endometrium. In particular, focus will be on the mid-secretory endometrium and appropriate markers and hormonal environment for successful implantation. This will be put in the context of the luteal phase of ovulation and the hormonal support that progesterone provides. We will also review pathologic states, such as endometriosis and related progesterone resistance, which affect mid-secretory phase and implantation. Finally, we will provide a detailed review of the literature on what the current state of knowledge is regarding receptivity and the microenvironment of the mid-secretory endometrium which is essential to implantation.

**Keywords:** secretory, implantation

## 1. Introduction

The female reproductive system prepares women for conception and pregnancy through two distinct, but highly integrated, cycles, the ovarian cycle and the endometrial cycle. The human endometrium, under the influence of complex biological signals, undergoes cyclic changes in preparation for implantation and the initiation of pregnancy. An array of molecular activity, still poorly understood, gives rise to relatively consistent morphologic changes of the endometrium during each cycle. In an era of assisted reproductive technologies (ART), there exists an ever-increasing demand to delineate these pathways in order to improve pregnancy rates. Ultimately, success in the field of reproduction and fertility requires an understanding of these complex processes, from molecular to cellular to tissue, in both the healthy patient as well as in the setting of various pathologic states.

This chapter will discuss the endometrial cycle with an emphasis on the secretory phase, including the molecular and biochemical components of endometrial receptivity and implantation. Markers and techniques for assessment of receptivity will be reviewed, as well as pathologic states that alter fertility.

## 2. The menstrual cycle and the endometrium

The endometrium is comprised of two anatomic layers, the functionalis and the basalis. The functionalis is made up of a compact zone, including stroma underneath the luminal epithelium, and a spongy zone which lies above the basalis layer [1, 2]. It is the functionalis layer that is shed in the monthly menses. The basalis layer lies on the myometrium; it undergoes fewer cyclic changes compared to the functionalis layer and is responsible for regenerating the functionalis after menstruation (**Figure 1**).

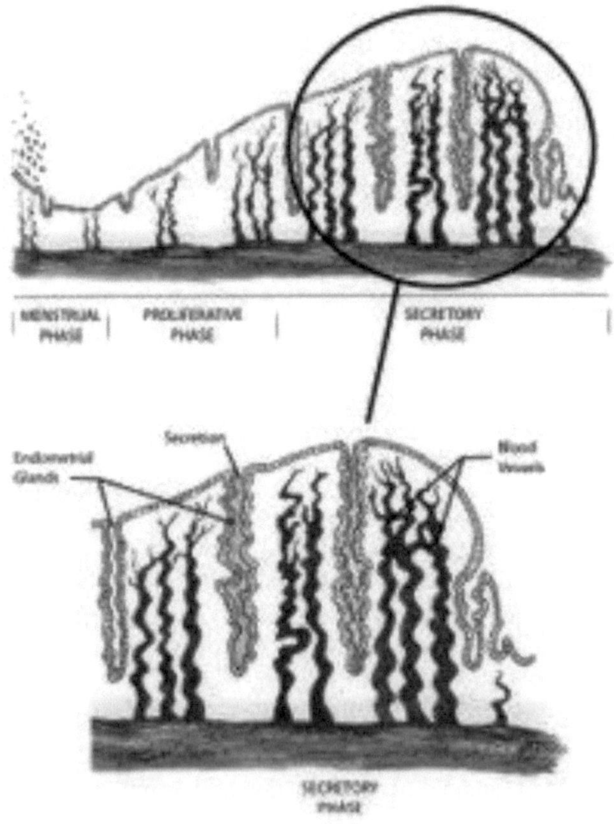


**Figure 1.** Functional anatomy of the human endometrium during the secretory phase.

The endometrial cycle consists of three sequential phases—the proliferative phase, secretory phase, and menstruation. Each phase is marked by physiologic changes that are controlled by circulating levels of estrogen and progesterone, which are synthesized and secreted from the ovary. The ovarian cycle is characterized by follicular development mediated by FSH (follicular phase), oocyte release mediated by the LH surge (ovulation), and development of the corpus luteum and production of progesterone (luteal phase). In the idealized 28-day cycle, ovulation occurs on day 14. After ovulation, the remnant of the dominant follicle becomes the corpus luteum, a temporary endocrine structure which produces progesterone (**Figure 1**) [1–4]. The corpus luteum becomes atretic on day 28 and menses begins the next day, establishing day 1 of the subsequent cycle.

During the proliferative phase, estradiol derived from the growing follicles drives the restoration of the functionalis layer with re-epithelialization by approximately day 5 of the menstrual cycle. This phase is characterized by hypertrophy and proliferation of glands, increase in stromal matrix, and elongation of terminal arterioles to the endometrial lumen. A gradient of angiogenic factors, particularly VEGF, is released from the endometrial epithelium by estradiol [5]. Estrogen also upregulates the progesterone receptors that orchestrate the environment during the secretory phase, which will be covered in more detail in the next section [2, 4]. In the absence of fertilization, progesterone levels decline due to atresia of the corpus luteum. This leads to vasospasm, ischemia, subsequent tissue death and endometrial shedding, or menses.

## 3. The secretory phase

For decades, endometrial dating has been assessed histologically [4, 6]. After ovulation, there is an increase in superficial stromal edema that becomes generalized by day 21. Stromal cells near terminal spiral arteries show an increase in cytoplasmic volume and surrounding extracellular matrix, a process termed predecidualization, which eventually encompasses the majority of the superficial endometrium by day 25. This transformation appears to represent a form of mesenchymal-to-epithelial transition (MET) [7]. By day 27, the superficial stromal cells are nearly indistinguishable from decidual cells of pregnancy. The increasing edema during the secretory phase results in the global endometrial thickening that is readily apparent with ultrasonography. Throughout the secretory phase, there are also distinct changes in spiral arteries. They rapidly lengthen, outpacing endometrial thickening, and become increasingly coiled [4, 6, 8, 9].

During the proliferative phase, there is an increase in glandular epithelium mitotic activity and pseudostratification of nuclei. There is a parallel increase in the proliferation of stromal components as well during this phase. After ovulation, this process is replaced by secretory transformation of glands and a slowing of stromal proliferation. At the cellular level, the early-secretory phase glands are characterized by abundant endoplasmic reticulum, accumulation of glycogen-rich vacuoles, and displacement of nuclei centrally. Six days after ovulation, loss of vacuoles from the cytoplasm corresponds with maximal glandular secretory activity [4, 9].

A complex interplay between mesenchymal cells and immune cells highlights the secretory phase of the superficial endometrial stroma. A substantial portion of the uterine leukocyte population is made up of CD56–/CD16+ uterine natural killer (uNK) cells, which are believed to play a tolerizing role in maternal allorecognition of fetal trophoblasts, rather than cytotoxicity. This cell population increases dramatically after ovulation and vanishes before menses in the absence of pregnancy. When conception occurs, the uNK cells are largely found in proximity to spiral arteries and extravillous trophoblasts in early pregnancy. The activity of uNK cells have been shown to be controlled by steroid hormones as well as local chemokines, including those containing the (C-X-C motif) and various interleukins [1, 4].

Macrophages (CD68+ and CD163+) are also found in the superficial endometrium, rapidly accumulating in the stroma after ovulation and declining in the absence of progesterone. T cells are found scattered throughout the endometrium with little to no menstrual-cycle change in concentration, as well as uterine dendritic cells (uDCs) which are most prominent in decidua of pregnancy [4].

The end of the secretory phase and beginning of the premenstrual phase is characterized by degradation of the stromal network, infiltration of the stroma by leukocytes, and cessation of glandular activity in the absence of the appropriate signals, such as hCG from developing trophectoderm. The degradation of the stromal network is catalyzed by matrix metalloproteinases (MMP), which become activated in the setting of falling progesterone levels. Evidence of apoptosis is evident throughout the tissue, and the ultrastructurally electron-dense contents of glandular cells characteristic of secretion vanish. These structures include the well-developed rough endoplasmic reticulum, Golgi apparatus, and glycogen-secreting cytoplasmic projections [1, 4].

## 4. Microarchitecture and implantation

The implantation of the blastocyst is a highly organized, selective process that, with some variations, is preserved among mammals. In women, nonhuman primates and other hemochorial placental species a narrow "window of implantation" (WOI) exists, during which the endometrium is capable of "receiving" the trophectoderm of the blastocyst. The interaction is orchestrated by a variety of molecules and is overall regulated by steroid hormones [4, 9]. Recent research suggests the WOI only lasts between 12 and 48 h, and is often shifted in patients with infertility [3]. In 1999, Wilcox et al. narrowed the timing of implantation to between 8 and 10 days after ovulation, with increased embryonic losses correlated with later implantation [10].

The process of implantation follows four well-described steps, which is coordinated with endometrial preparation by changes in steroid hormones. The focus here starts with apposition and transient adhesion of syncytial trophoblast cells to the endometrial epithelium, which is followed by firm attachment and finally, trophoblast invasion. As the blastocyst enters the uterine cavity, the zona pellucida is shed allowing for exposure of the trophectoderm [9, 11]. Driven by progesterone, the secretory phase endometrial epithelial cells enter a hypersecretory state, with characteristic features described as the *Arias-Stella reaction*. This hypersecretory state of the tissue provides the necessary histiotrophic nutrition essential for embryo and placental survival, as vascular remodeling occurs later [12, 13].

The molecular basis of blastocyst invasion is of active interest in the field, as failure of these mechanisms is associated with pregnancy loss. Current research suggests that mucin (MUC)1, a large transmembrane mucin and a barrier to implantation is downregulated and/or removed through the action of surface proteases and decreased expression of progesterone receptors. The loss of MUC1 allows for appropriate apposition, adhesion, and attachment of the embryo to the endometrium. Initial transient adhesion is mediated by selectins and galectins. More firm attachment is mediated by integrins, including $\alpha\nu\beta3$ and $\alpha4\beta1$, and CD44 and their shared ligand, osteopontin (OPN). Other attachment-associated molecules include trophinin, HB-EGF, fibronectin, vitronectin, laminin, IGFBP1, and the latency associated peptide linked to TGFβ [2–4, 9, 11].

Specialized surface macromolecules have also been implicated in blastocyst adhesion and invasion. Endometrial epithelium consists of both ciliated and nonciliated, secretory cells, the proportions of which are regulated by estrogen levels. The secretory cells develop transient surface structures in response to progesterone levels, called pinopodes, during the time of maximal receptivity [14]. These structures are involved in pinocytosis and contain various adhesion molecules, including $\alpha\nu\beta3$, glycodelin, and OPN [15]. The development of pinopodes is dependent upon HOXA-10, a homeobox gene whose expression is vital for endometrial receptivity, regulating both endometrial stromal cell proliferation and epithelial cell morphogenesis [16]. Blocking the expression of HOXA-10 results in a significant reduction in the number of pinopodes. Although some evidence points to pinopodes role in adhesion and invasion of the embryo, their precise function and overall importance is still debated [2, 3].

Adhesion via these molecules is static dynamic process. Extracellular contact with appropriate ligands transmits signals, through a variety of pathways, into intracellular cascades that results in gene transcription and protein expression that mediate migration, proliferation, and cytoskeletal remodeling. The overall result is the successful invasion of the embryo into a primed endometrium, where it has the potential for growth and development [2–4].

## 5. Receptivity markers and clinical applications

The assessment of endometrial receptivity has drastically changed since the establishment of the Noyes' criteria for histologic dating in 1950 [6]. Once the clinical significance of the pathological criteria was questioned, a more detailed understanding of the biochemical pathways influenced by steroid hormones during the menstrual cycle led to new targets to identify endometrial receptivity [17]. Initially, single molecules were analyzed. With the advent of microarray technology and massively parallel, next generation RNA sequencing, vast amounts of molecules can be analyzed at the same time to give a much more complete picture of the endometrial environment [1, 3, 4].

Cytokines are involved in many processes of the ovarian and endometrial cycles and have been shown to play a critical role in implantation. Leukemia inhibitory factor (LIF) is an IL-6 family member and its expression has been demonstrated in the human endometrial epithelium during the mid- to late-secretory phase [16]. In women of proven fertility, endometrial biopsies demonstrated LIF mRNA expression increased from day 18 to 28, with a peak at day 20, and showed a corresponding 2.2-fold increase in LIF protein secretion between the proliferative and secretory phase [18]. IL-6, another cytokine expressed in the endometrium shows a regulated temporal pattern throughout the menstrual cycle with the highest detected levels during the luteal phase. IL-6 mRNA levels increase progressively during the mid- to late-secretory phase and IL-6 protein was strongly expressed in luminal and glandular epithelial cells during the window of implantation. The protein is strongly pronounced. Bone morphogenic protein 2 (BMP2), a member of the TGF-β superfamily, is first detected in the stroma surrounding the site of blastocyst attachment during the mid-secretory phase. BMP2 is considered a critical regulator of decidualization due to its role in regulating proliferation and differentiation, as well as its expression during the implantation period [19, 20].

Amniotic fluid contains very high concentrations (~5 μg/ml) of prolactin (PRL), which is produced by the decidua. It has been determined that endometrial PRL production begins around cycle day 22, and levels rise throughout pregnancy. Similarly, high levels of IGFBP-1 and LEFTY2 are produced by secretory phase endometrium in response to progesterone and expression of these can be recapitulated in vitro. Given their abundance and production during the menstrual cycle, these proteins serve as potential markers for endometrial receptivity, although clinic utility is not yet clear [1–4, 11].

Prostaglandins (PGs) have been shown to play a crucial role for successful embryo implantation due to their vasoactive properties. The generation of PGs from membrane-bound arachidonic acid is achieved by cytosolic phospholipase $A_2$ ($cPLA_2$) and cyclooxygenase (COX). Studies in female mice lacking $cPLA_2$ or COX-2 enzymes have demonstrated the vital role of PGs in implantation. $PGE_2$ and $PGF_{2\alpha}$ expression was detected in human endometrium throughout all stages of the menstrual cycle but was downregulated during the late-secretory phase [16].

Several integrins have been identified as possible markers of uterine receptivity and have been noted to undergo alterations in the epithelium and decidua during implantation. The co-expression of α1β1, ανβ3, and α4β1 heterodimers marks the period of endometrial receptivity by mediating firm attachment between the embryo and endometrium. The regulated expression of secretory phase integrins suggests that steroid hormones likely play a role in their presence; for example, α1β1/laminin receptor (VLA-1) expression on secretory phase endometrial epithelium is suggestive of progesterone-induced upregulation. The firm attachment mediated by integrins also generates other integrin-associated ligands. OPN, a ligand for ανβ3, is significantly upregulation in endometrial epithelial cells and mediates cellular adhesion and migration during embryo implantation. Calcitonin, a known upregulator of ανβ3, is transiently produced in the uterine epithelia during the period of implantation. It downregulates E-cadherin expression and promotes the outgrowth of trophoblasts into the uterus [16, 21].

Another critical endometrial glycoprotein, MUC1, is a factor that interferes with cellular adhesion. MUC1 is likely the first uterine molecule that the blastocyst encounters during the apposition phase, where it is thought to repel the embryo until the time and place is ideal for firm attachment. This is confirmed by the apparent local downregulation of MUC1 by progesterone before implantation in the receptive endometrium of mice. The reduced expression facilitates embryo-epithelial interactions by unmasking cell adhesion molecules on the endometrial surface [16]. When measured in humans, MUC1 showed increased generalized expression during the peri-implantation period, somewhat contradicting the studies in other species.

Two cytoskeleton-related proteins, stathmin 1 and annexin A2, have opposing regulation in the receptive versus pre-receptive endometrium. Stathmin 1 is a phosphoprotein that regulates microtubule dynamics during cell cycle progression, specifically at the embryo implantation site. In receptive human endometrium, downregulation of stathmin 1 supports decidualization. Annexin A2, an apical surface molecule in receptive human endometrium, is involved in cellular differentiation, regulation of prolactin secretion, and prostaglandin formation. Annexin A2 expression is highest in the mid- to late-secretory phase and decreased in the pre-receptive phase. This pattern of expression, along with in vitro effects on embryo adhesiveness, suggests annexin A2 plays a role in implantation [22].

BCL6, a transcriptional repressor mutated in some lymphomas, is associated with inflammation and significantly elevated values are seen in the secretory phase of patients with endometriosis and otherwise unexplained infertility. Data suggest that BCL6 is associated with progesterone resistance, leading to implantation defects and increased IVF failures [23, 24]. It is being developed as a diagnostic biomarker for endometriosis.

Ion channels and gap junctions in the endometrium have recently demonstrated a role in regulating endometrial receptivity and embryo implantation. The volume of electrolyte-containing fluid in the uterine lumen fluctuates throughout the menstrual cycle under the influence of ovarian hormones and is significantly reduced in the mid-secretory phase, encouraging blastocyst-endometrial apposition. This is suggestive of a net fluid absorption across the endometrium during the receptive phase. Cystic fibrosis transmembrane conductance regulator (CFTR) mediates $Cl^-$ efflux, which is essential for epithelial fluid secretion. The endometrial epithelium is known to contain CFTR, playing an active role in endometrial $Cl^-$ and fluid secretion. Downregulation of CFTR by progesterone during the secretory phase contributes to the decrease in fluid volume, which aids embryo implantation. The epithelial sodium channel (ENaC) also is present in the endometrium establishing a sodium gradient and providing a driving force for water absorption. CFTR has an inhibitory effect on ENaC, so the downregulation of CFTR during the secretory phase enhances the absorptive activity of the endometrial epithelium. ENaC is upregulated by progesterone, furthering the absorptive properties of the endometrial epithelium during the secretory phase. Other ion channels such as $K^+$ and $Ca^{2+}$ and ion transporters, SLC4 and SLC26, are emerging as important players in regulating certain processes of embryo implantation [19]. Connexin 43 gap junctions also appear to mediate water and small molecule (<1.2 nm Stokes radius) transport and decidual differentiation [7, 25].

Microarray analysis of endometrial tissue allows for assessment of hundreds to thousands of molecules at once. Genomic and proteomic analyses have identified varying levels of genes and proteins implicated in a wide array of activities during decidualization. Receptivity markers are measured in clinical settings to avoid implantation failure and to hopefully provide a more favorable outcome for patients utilizing ART. Although some of the mentioned biomarkers have only recently been discovered as key players in the human receptive endometrium, these discoveries show promise in better understanding the complex interactions throughout the secretory phase and window of implantation.

Aspiration and assessment of secreted uterine fluids, called secretomics, which largely looks at protein and lipid levels, allows for high-throughput analysis of endometrial secretions during the secretory phase without the need for biopsies. Although our understanding of microarray technology as it related to infertility is still evolving, current and future products on the market will likely find clinical utility and are discussed in more detail later in the chapter [3, 26, 27].

## 6. Pathologic states and the secretory phase

Given the complex nature of endometrial receptivity, it is very vulnerable to perturbation. Local factors that can negatively impact receptivity and implantation can be broadly grouped into mechanical and inflammatory factors. Mechanical abnormalities encompass both congenital anomalies and acquired conditions. Local inflammatory factors include endometriosis, adenomyosis, hydrosalpinges, and endometritis [2, 28, 29].

Mechanical abnormalities of the uterus such as uterine septa, fibroids, polyps, and adhesions result in physical barriers to successful fertilization and implantation. These conditions are linked with recurrent pregnancy loss and infertility and substantial evidence exists that shows surgical correction of these abnormalities can improve outcomes [2, 29].

Given the delicate regulation of the menstrual cycle and the narrow implantation window, inflammatory factors that affect signaling pathways can effectively derail normal physiologic processes. In the setting of local inflammation, progesterone resistance and estrogen receptor dominance can result in impaired implantation. With endometriosis, for instance, there is an increase in inflammatory cytokines including TNF$\alpha$, INF$\gamma$, IL-1, and IL-17. This leads to downstream effects such as phosphorylated STAT3, which in turn leads to an estrogen dominant and progesterone resistant state, shown through microarray analysis [2, 28]. Decreased expression of IL-11 and CCL4, which are associated with embryo receptivity, is found in chronic endometritis and is believed to be related to infertility associated with this condition [30]. Low integrin levels have been associated with inflammatory conditions and reduced $\alpha\nu\beta3$ expression, which can be caused by increased estrogen levels, and have been tied to IVF failure. Conversely, aromatase overexpression is seen in inflammatory states, and is linked with predicting failure in ART cycles. Other chemokines and cytokines, such as interleukins, are similarly linked to inflammation and pregnancy failure [2].

Although there still exist many gaps in our understanding of endometrial receptivity and implantation at the level of the uterus, pregnancy and ART failure cannot be fully explained by local factors. There exist several systemic disorders that can impact the uterine environment and the embryo's ability to implant. These diseases include thyroid dysfunction, vitamin D deficiency, hyperprolactinemia, inflammatory bowel disease, obesity, and smoking. There exists significant evidence relating hypothyroidism and poor fertility/IVF success rates, prompting levothyroxine treatment in patients with TSH < 2.5 mIU/L [2]. Obesity has similarly been linked to infertility, with evidence demonstrating that even modest weight loss improves pregnancy rates [2, 31]. However, our understanding of how these systemic states affect fertility is still limited, and further research is warranted to fully evaluate these relationships.

## 7. Future directions

Historically, dating of the receptive endometrium was based on morphologic criteria [6]. Shortcomings in the sensitivity and specificity of this method, fueled by significant advances in our molecular understanding of the endometrial cycle, have led to new approaches [17]. Although utilization of single molecular markers has not yielded satisfactory results, high-throughput analysis has been more promising [3]. The recent application of the "-omics" technologies, that utilize high-throughput techniques with sophisticated large data analysis to generate far more detailed patterns of molecular and biochemical processes, has revolutionized our understanding of the receptive endometrium and promises to yield clinically useful tools [3, 4, 26, 27].

The analysis of the endometrial cycle using transcriptomics has been actively investigated for over a decade [3]. Using gene expression microarray techniques, researchers have been able to study the expression of thousands of genes simultaneously during different phases of the endometrial cycle. They have identified unique gene profiles during the window of implantation, which includes important factors previously identified, such as LIF, OPN, CXCL14, glycodelin, IL15, L-selectin ligands, and various antioxidants [3]. One example of a commercially successful diagnostic test based on a transcription signature is the endometrial receptivity array (ERA). In controlled trials, use of this tool identified shifted windows of implantation in women with implantation failure. Using the test to adjust the timing of embryo transfer yielded pregnancy and implantation rates similar to control groups [32].

Although the current transcriptomics method has yielded impressive results, it relies on a tissue biopsy. An alternative matrix that researchers have analyzed since the 1970s is endometrial fluid [16]. More recently, high-throughput analysis of vaginal secretions, coined secretomics, has been utilized [26, 33]. As it focuses on sampling extracellular fluid, the analytes of interest are mainly proteins and lipids, with mass spectroscopy and chromatography used as the analytical methods. Analysis of lipid levels has revealed elevated levels of PGE2 and PGF2α during the WOI. Although preliminary information from endometrial secretions is intriguing, further investigation is required [26, 33].

Our understanding of infertility and endometrial receptivity has come a long way over the past several decades. However, many questions remain unanswered. New molecular and biochemical markers during the endometrial cycle continue to be discovered and they are likely to inform even better diagnostic algorithms. These include potential targets for pharmaceuticals and predictors of therapeutic success. Discoveries in this arena are fueled by advances in research technologies. High-throughput analysis, in particular, has revolutionized the field. Massively parallel sequencing will allow an even more detailed look at the unique genomic and transcriptomic signatures of the receptive endometrium. Translation of this research into clinical trials, and then clinical practice, is expected to have a major impact on the field of reproductive endocrinology and infertility.

## Author details

Courtney Marsh[1]*, Katelyn Schumacher[2], Warren B. Nothnick[3,4,5], Robert N. Taylor[6] and Monique Monard[1]

*Address all correspondence to: cmarsh2@kumc.edu

1 Department of Obstetrics and Gynecology, University of Kansas, Kansas City, KS, USA

2 School of Medicine, University of Kansas, Kansas City, KS, USA

3 Department of Molecular and Integrative Physiology, University of Kansas Medical Center, Kansas City, Kansas, USA

4 Department of Obstetrics and Gynecology, University of Kansas Medical Center, Kansas City, Kansas, USA

5 Center for Reproductive Sciences, Institute for Reproduction and Perinatal Research, University of Kansas Medical Center, Kansas City, Kansas, USA

6 Department of Obstetrics and Gynecology, University of Utah, Salt Lake City, UT, USA

## References

[1] Critchley HO, Saunders PT. Hormone receptor dynamics in a receptive human endometrium. Reproductive Sciences. 2009;**16**(2):191-199

[2] Fox C, Morin S, Jeong JW, Scott RT Jr, Lessey BA. Local and systemic factors and implantation: What is the evidence? Fertility and Sterility. 2016;**105**(4):873-884

[3] Gómez E, Ruíz-Alonso M, Miravet J, Simón C. Human endometrial transcriptomics: Implications for embryonic implantation. Cold Spring Harbor Perspectives in Medicine. 2015;**5**(7):a022996

[4] Gellersen B, Brosens JJ. Cyclic decidualization of the human endometrium in reproductive health and failure. Endocrine Reviews. 2014;**35**(6):851-905

[5] Taylor RN, Lebovic DI, Hornung D, Mueller MD. Endocrine and paracrine regulation of endometrial angiogenesis. Annals of the New York Academy of Sciences. 2001;**943**: 109-121

[6] Noyes RW, Hertig AT, Rock J. Dating the endometrial biopsy. Fertility and Sterility. 1950;**1**:3-25

[7] Yu J, Berga SL, Johnston-MacAnanny EB, Sidell N, Bagchi IC, Bagchi MK, et al. Endometrial stromal decidualization responds reversibly to hormone stimulation and withdrawal. Endocrinology. 2016;**157**:2432-2446

[8] Rock J, Bartlett MK. Biopsy studies of human endometrium: Criteria of dating and information about amenorrhea, menorrhagia, and time of ovulation. Journal of the American Medical Association. 1937;**108**:2022-2028

[9] Bazer FW, Spencer TE, Johnson GA, Burghardt RC, Wu G. Comparative aspects of implantation. Reproduction. 2009;**138**(2):195-209

[10] Wilcox AJ, Baird DD, Weinberg CR. Time of implantation of the conceptus and loss of pregnancy. The New England Journal of Medicine. 1999;**340**(23):1796-1799

[11] Bazer FW, Wu G, Spencer TE, Johnson GA, Burghardt RC, Bayless K. Novel pathways for implantation and establishment and maintenance of pregnancy in mammals. Molecular Human Reproduction. 2010;**16**(3):135-152

[12] Arias-Stella J. The Arias-Stella reaction: Facts and fancies four decades after. Advances in Anatomic Pathology. 2002;**9**(1):12-23. Review

[13] Burton GJ, Watson AL, Hempstock J, Skepper JN, Jauniaux E. Uterine glands provide histiotrophic nutrition for the human fetus during the first trimester of pregnancy. The Journal of Clinical Endocrinology and Metabolism. 2002;**87**(6):2954-2959

[14] Nikas G, Psychoyos A. Uterine pinopodes in peri-implantation human endometrium. Clinical relevance. Annals of the New York Academy of Sciences. 1997;**816**:129-142. Review

[15] Stavreus-Evers A, Mandelin E, Koistinen R, Aghajanova L, Hovatta O, Seppälä M. Glycodelin is present in pinopodes of receptive-phase human endometrium and is associated with down-regulation of progesterone receptor B. Fertility and Sterility. 2006;**85**(6): 1803-1811

[16] Achache H, Revel A. Endometrial receptivity markers, the journey to successful embryo implantation. Human Reproduction Update. 2006;**12**(6):731-746

[17] Coutifaris C, Myers ER, Guzick DS, Diamond MP, Carson SA, Legro RS, et al. Histological dating of timed endometrial biopsy tissue is not related to fertility status. Fertility and Sterility. 2004;**82**(5):1264-1272

[18] Garrido-Gómez T, Quiñonero A, Antúnez O, Díaz-Gimeno P, Bellver J, Simón C, et al. Deciphering the proteomic signature of human endometrial receptivity. Human Reproduction. 2014;**29**(9):1957-1967

[19] Ruan YC, Chen H, Chan HC. Ion channels in the endometrium: Regulation of endometrial receptivity and embryo implantation. Human Reproduction Update. 2014;**20**(4):517-529

[20] Li Q, Kannan A, Wang W, Demayo FJ, Taylor RN, Bagchi MK, et al. Bone morphogenetic protein 2 functions via a conserved signaling pathway involving Wnt4 to regulate uterine

decidualization in the mouse and the human. The Journal of Biological Chemistry. 2007;**282**(43):31725-31732

[21] Lessey BA. Endometrial integrins and the establishment of uterine receptivity. Human Reproduction. 1998;**13**(Suppl_3):247-258

[22] Dominguez F, Garrido-Gomez T, Lopez JA, Camafeita E, Quinonero A, Pellicer A, et al. Proteomic analysis of the human receptive versus non-receptive endometrium using differential in-gel electrophoresis and MALDI-MS unveils stathmin 1 and annexin A2 as differentially regulated. Human Reproduction. 2009;**24**(10):2607-2617

[23] Evans-Hoeker E, Lessey BA, Jeong JW, Savaris RF, Palomino WA, Yuan L, et al. Endometrial BCL6 overexpression in eutopic endometrium of women with endometriosis. Reproductive Sciences. 2016;**23**(9):1234-1241

[24] Miravet-Valenciano JA, Rincon-Bertolin A, Vilella F, Simon C. Understanding and improving endometrial receptivity. Current Opinion in Obstetrics and Gynecology. 2015;**27**(3): 187-192

[25] Matson BC, Pierce SL, Espenschied ST, Holle E, Sweatt IH, Davis ES, et al. Adrenomedullin improves fertility and promotes pinopodes and cell junctions in the peri-implantation endometrium. Biology of Reproduction. 2017;**97**(3):466-477

[26] Berlanga O, Bradshaw HB, Vilella-Mitjana F, Garrido-Gómez T, Simón C. How endometrial secretomics can help in predicting implantation. Placenta. 2011;**32**(Suppl. 3): S271-S275

[27] Díaz-Gimeno P, Ruíz-Alonso M, Blesa D, Simón C. Transcriptomics of the human endometrium. The International Journal of Developmental Biology. 2014;**58**(2-4):127-137

[28] Ahn SH, Singh V, Tayade C. Biomarkers in endometriosis: Challenges and opportunities. Fertility and Sterility. 2017;**107**(3):523-532

[29] Revel A. Defective endometrial receptivity. Fertility and Sterility. 2012;**97**(5):1028-1032

[30] Kitaya K, Matsubayashi H, Yamaguchi K, Nishiyama R, Takaya Y, Ishikawa T, et al. Chronic endometritis: Potential cause of infertility and obstetric and neonatal complications. American Journal of Reproductive Immunology. 2016;**75**(1):13-22

[31] Marsh CA, Hecker E. Maternal obesity and adverse reproductive outcomes: Reducing the risk. Obstetrical & Gynecological Survey. 2014;**69**(10):622-628

[32] Díaz-Gimeno P, Horcajadas JA, Martínez-Conejero JA, Esteban FJ, Alamá P, Pellicer A, et al. A genomic diagnostic tool for human endometrial receptivity based on the transcriptomic signature. Fertility and Sterility. 2011;**95**(1):50-60. 60.e1-15

[33] Cheong Y, Boomsma C, Heijnen C, Macklon N. Uterine secretomics: A window on the maternal-embryo interface. Fertility and Sterility. 2013;**99**(4):1093-1099

Chapter 5

# Menstrual Cycle and Physical Effort

Magdalena Wiecek

Additional information is available at the end of the chapter

http://dx.doi.org/10.5772/intechopen.79675

**Abstract**

In addition to affecting the sexual organs in women, ovarian hormones have a wide impact on processes related to metabolism, water and electrolyte balance, thermoregulation, and redox balance. Differences in the estradiol and progesterone concentrations during the follicular and luteal phases, as well as the increase in the concentration of these hormones under the influence of physical exercise, may cause a different course of exercise response in women depending on the phase of menstrual cycle. Estrogens affect the metabolism of women by reducing the rate of gluconeogenesis and glycogenolysis and, at the same time, by increasing the share of lipids in covering energy requirements. Progesterone affects respiratory system parameters causing, among others, an increase in pulmonary ventilation. The resultant antagonistic action of progesterone and estradiol is the effect on thermoregulatory mechanisms. Increased estradiol concentration at the low progesterone concentration level causes water and electrolyte retention. In turn, an increased level of progesterone leads to loss of water and sodium, causing a decrease in the volume of plasma during the postovulatory phase of the menstrual cycle. The processes described above are related to metabolic changes affecting the ability to perform physical efforts.

**Keywords:** menstrual cycle, aerobic efforts, anaerobic efforts, acid-base balance, redox balance

## 1. Introduction

Knowledge about the physiology of physical efforts is mostly based on research results in which only men participated. However, the increasing participation of women in many sports disciplines encourages observation of the physiological reactions and effects regarding intense physical efforts on the body of women associated with the process of sports training [1, 2].

A decrease in the level of sex hormones during rest, as a result of heavy and long-term training, can lead to disorders in the menstrual cycle of a woman [2, 3]. These disorders most have the characteristics of rare menstrual periods (oligomenorrhea) or secondary amenorrhea (amenorrhoea secundaria). In women with regular menstruation, burdened by sports training, anovulatory cycles or shortened luteal phases often occur. It is also possible to exclude the impact of physical exercise related to training on the later menarche age [2, 4]. The factors conducive to hormonal abnormalities are large decreases in body mass and the amount of adipose tissue, resulting not only from significant training loads but also frequent disorders in the way of eating [5]. Long-lasting estrogen deficiency leads to a decrease in bone density, causing deterioration of its structure, which may contribute to osteoporosis in the future [6]. Abnormalities in the way of eating, menstrual disorders, and disturbances in bone metabolism observed in women practicing various sports were called the "triad syndrome" [2, 7, 8]. Therefore, one should look for an answer to the question on how to program women's training in order to achieve high sports results without negative consequences for their health [1].

Assessing physiological responses induced by physical exercise in women, cyclic changes in the level of sex hormones that occur during the reproductive period in every normal menstrual cycle cannot be overlooked. The menstrual cycle is the result of complex interaction of the hypothalamus, pituitary gland, and ovarian hormones, which, apart from acting on the sexual organs, exhibit a broad, nonspecific effect on various processes related to metabolism, water, and electrolyte balance or thermoregulation in women [2, 9–13]. As shown in studies on animals, differences related to estradiol levels are a factor influencing the diversified use of energy substrates [14, 15]. Distinct differences in estradiol and progesterone levels between the follicular and luteal phases, as well as an increase in the concentration of these hormones under the influence of physical exercise, may cause a different course of exercise response in women depending on the phase of the menstrual cycle [2, 10, 16].

Research suggests that estrogens affect the metabolism of women by reducing the rate of gluconeogenesis and glycogenolysis and, at the same time, increase the share of lipids in covering energy demand [17–22]. The increased use of lipids as a source of energy occurs due to the increase in the amount of free fatty acids, which results from the increased synthesis of triglycerides and in the rate of lipolysis [23]. The effect of estradiol on metabolic processes in the liver, muscles, and adipose tissue can be achieved by changing the activity of key enzymes, changing membrane permeability or indirectly through changes in hormone levels: insulin, glucagon, cortisol, hGH, or catecholamines [24, 25].

Progesterone affects the parameters of the respiratory system, causing, inter alia, an increase in pulmonary ventilation per minute ($V_E$) [26]. In the postovulatory phase, a higher resting level of oxygen uptake ($VO_2$) is also observed [27].

The resultant antagonistic effect of progesterone and estradiol is the effect on thermoregulatory mechanisms, which leads to an increase in the body's core temperature during the luteal phase of the menstrual cycle [12, 28–30].

In the woman's body, we also observe changes in the total water content associated with the menstrual cycle phase. Observations of some authors indicate that elevated estradiol concentration at low concentration of progesterone causes the retention of water and electrolytes in the body [31]. In turn, the increased level of progesterone, by blocking the action of aldosterone in the kidneys, leads to loss of water and sodium [32], causing a decrease in plasma volume during the postovulatory phase of the menstrual cycle [33].

All processes described above are directly related to metabolic changes affecting the ability to perform physical efforts. Differences in the use of substrates and in the intensity of individual energy changes during muscle work of different intensities, resulting from hormonal changes in the course of the menstrual cycle, may affect, e.g., the activity of the adrenergic system, the amount of lactic acid formed in muscle tissue and its level in the blood, and changes in the level of acid-base balance parameters or indicators of oxidative stress [2, 10, 16, 34]. Therefore, it can be expected that cyclical fluctuations in the level of endogenous ovarian hormones in women will affect the extent and size of exercise responses. However, the test results are not unequivocal.

## 2. Methods

Original and review scientific publications regarding the level of cardiopulmonary reactions, thermoregulation processes, and oxidative stress as a result of aerobic and anaerobic efforts during various phases of the menstrual cycle were reviewed. Conclusions were formulated on the basis of tests in which hormonal evaluation of the menstrual cycle was conducted.

## 3. Exercise responses during the menstrual cycle

### 3.1. Aerobic exercise

It is generally accepted that the maximal oxygen uptake index ($VO_{2max}$) is the indicator of aerobic efficiency, the level of which is directly determined during gradual physical exercise, performed up to the individual maximum intensity ("until exhaustion"). Such effort leads to the maximum involvement of the oxidative phosphorylation process while activating the processes of anaerobic adenosine triphosphate (ATP) resynthesis (phosphocreatine, anaerobic glycolysis). VE, cardiac output, and blood oxygen capacity are important factors determining the level of $VO_{2max}$ [35].

#### *3.1.1. Cardiorespiratory effect*

One of the first studies comparing the physiological and biochemical stress response of women at the time of the menstrual cycle, during which laboratory testing days were determined based on sex hormone levels, was carried out by Jurkowski et al. [36]. In these studies, immediately after two 20-minute physical efforts at an intensity of 40 and 70% $VO_{2max}$, respectively, the woman performed a physical effort at an intensity of 90% $VO_{2max}$ "until exhaustion." The time of extreme exercise was almost twice as long in the luteal phase. In the luteal phase, higher values of the maximum minute pulmonary ventilation ($VE_{max}$) were also noted. The maximum heart rate ($HR_{max}$) and $VO_{2max}$ did not differ between the menstrual cycle phases [36].

However, these data are not fully confirmed in the results of research conducted by other authors. The time of continuing the effort of gradually increasing work intensity did not differ significantly between the follicular and luteal phases of the menstrual cycle [37]. Similar in both phases of the menstrual cycle, Nicklas et al. [17] found that the time of continuing work "until exhaustion " was for the intensity of 70% $VO_{2max}$, and McCracken et al. [38] noted it for the intensity of 90% $VO_{2max}$.

The results of some studies indicate a significantly higher level of resting oxygen uptake during the postovulatory phase [27, 39]. However, most authors agree that the menstrual cycle phases do not significantly affect $VO_2$, neither at rest nor during submaximal and maximal intensity efforts [37, 40–45].

The conclusions from laboratory tests differ regarding the assessment of the influence of the menstrual cycle phases on the level of pulmonary ventilation. Schoene et al. [46] and Das [47] reported higher resting $V_E$ values in the luteal phase of the menstrual cycle. During stress tests, Jurkowski et al. [36], as well as Hessemer and Bruck [39], obtained higher values in the postovulatory phase. However, differences between phases in the exercise level of this parameter are not statistically significant in many studies [37, 43, 45, 48].

Significant inter-phase differences concerning the maximal heart rate were noted by Pivarnik et al. [41]. In this research, $HR_{max}$ was higher in the luteal phase by 10 beats per minute. Higher resting and exercise heart rate in the luteal phase were also noted by other researchers [39, 46, 49]. Some authors, however, did not find significant differences in the values of $HR_{max}$ [37, 40, 43, 45, 48].

De Souza et al. [48], comparing the physiological responses of women with normal menstrual cycles and women with secondary menstrual irregularities, obtained similar results for both groups. In eumenorrheic women, both during the 40-minute effort at 80% intensity $VO_{2max}$ and during the graded test "until exhaustion," in the luteal phase, slightly higher levels of oxygen uptake, pulmonary ventilation, and heart rate were found. However, the postexercise concentration of lactate in the blood was lower in this phase. Nevertheless, the differences between phases were not statistically significant [48].

### *3.1.2. Metabolic effect*

It is undisputed that a gradual increase in the intensity of effort leads to an increase in anaerobic energy recovery processes. This causes an increase in the concentration of lactic acid in the blood, causing changes in the level of acid-base balance parameters [50–52]. Therefore, it is of great importance in the assessment of endurance capacities to determine the location of metabolic thresholds, using blood lactate measurement or based on the dynamics of changes in ventilation indicators. The first metabolic threshold is defined by the first ventilatory threshold, the aerobic or anaerobic threshold (AT), and means the addition of anaerobic metabolism. The second metabolic threshold is referred to as the second ventilatory threshold, respiratory compensation point (RCP), or the threshold of uncompensated metabolic acidosis [50, 52–55]. The severity of anaerobic transformation after exceeding this threshold causes hyperventilation and leads to the development of fatigue induced by incomplete metabolic acidosis [52, 56].

The results of many studies indicate the lack of clear influence of the menstrual cycle phases on resting and postexercise levels of lactate and acid-base balance parameters in the blood [17, 37, 43, 48, 57, 58].

One of the studies [45], during which women performed a graded test, indicated lower blood lactate and lower respiratory exchange ratio (RER) values for submaximal loads in the luteal phase. Resting levels and maximum values of blood lactate concentration did not significantly differ in both phases of the menstrual cycle [45]. Significantly, higher levels of lactate in the follicular phase were found by Lavoie et al. [59] during a 90-minute effort at intensity of approximately 63% $VO_{2max}$. Similar results were obtained by Jurkowski et al. [36] during an effort of 90% intensity $VO_{2max}$ and McCracken et al. [38] during a graded test. The authors found a statistically significant, higher level of resting blood lactate concentration in the follicular phase of the menstrual cycle. Also, increases in lactate concentration and decreases in buffering bases, after efforts with higher loads, were significantly greater in the follicular phase than the luteal phase [36]. Differences between phases in the postexercise lactate level were maintained for 30 minutes of restitution [38].

The purpose of the Devries et al.'s study [60] was, among others, to determine the effect of menstrual cycle phase upon glucose turnover and muscle glycogen utilization during moderate-intensity endurance exercise. In these studies, healthy, recreationally active young women underwent a primed constant infusion of glucose with muscle biopsies taken before and after a 90-minute cycling exercise at intensity of 65% $VO_{2max}$. In the studies, it was demonstrated that women in the luteal phase have lesser reliance on carbohydrate sources to fuel endurance exercise compared with follicular phase. It was evidenced by a lower glucose rate of appearance and disappearance as well as metabolic clearance rate and lower glycogen utilization during and at the end of exercise [60].

Higher oxidation of lipids and lower oxidation of carbohydrates in the luteal phase during submaximal efforts at an intensity higher than 50% $VO_{2max}$ have also been demonstrated in other studies [61–63]. It was also noticed that interphase differences in the use of energy substrates are related to the effort intensity. During a 30-minute treadmill run, healthy, well-menstruating women performed three 10-minute efforts at the following intensities: 30, 60, and 75% $VO_{2max}$, successively. Higher lipid oxidation in the luteal phase was found during low- and moderate-intensity exercise, while there were no interphase differences during exercise at an intensity of 75% $VO_{2max}$ [20]. Similar results were obtained that in cycling efforts, higher lipid oxidation in the luteal phase was found at the 30% intensity $VO_{2max}$ and 50% $VO_{2max}$, but not at 70% $VO_{2max}$ [64]. On the other hand, they are not confirmed by this study, in which, on the basis of RER, there were no differences between phases in the proportions of energy substrate consumption (lipids/carbohydrates) during efforts of a wide intensity range, i.e., 45% $VO_{2max}$ [65], 50% $VO_{2max}$ [66], 65% $VO_{2max}$ [65], 70% $VO_{2max}$ [67], as well as 80% $VO_{2max}$ [48].

Later research [68], in which young female rowers (female athletes and women practicing recreationally and taking/not taking oral contraceptive pills) performed a graded test on a rowing ergometer during the follicular and luteal phases of the menstrual cycle, showed that there are no interphase differences in the level of power output, ventilator equivalents of $O_2$ ($V_E/VO_2$), HR, and blood lactate concentration at maximal and aerobic-anaerobic transition intensities in all three groups. However, higher values were observed for ventilatory equivalents of $CO_2$ ($V_E/VCO_2$) at both intensities in the luteal phase compared with the follicular phase in the group of women taking contraceptive pills [68]. There were no significant interphase differences in the oxidation of carbohydrates and fats during resting (before the exercise) or during the 1-hour rowing exercise at 70% $VO_{2max}$. Energy expenditure, oxygen uptake, HR, and lactate concentration were similar in the follicular and luteal phases during this exercise [69]. In both phases of the menstrual cycle, the female rowers obtained similar values of $VO_{2max}$ and $VO_2$ at the threshold of anaerobic transitions [69]. These results are consistent with those previously presented by Smekal et al. [70], who showed that there are no significant intergroup differences in the level of power output, $VO_2$, RER, HR, and blood lactate concentration at rest, at maximal load, and at different thresholds of aerobic and anaerobic metabolism (lactate thresholds, respiratory thresholds: AT and RCP), which were measured during a cycle test in eumenorrheic women. In this study, minute ventilation and $V_E/VO_2$ and $V_E/VCO_2$ indices were higher in the luteal phase at rest, exhaustion, and AT [70].

#### *3.1.3. Oxygen capacity of the blood*

Another important factor determining the level of $VO_{2max}$ is the oxygen capacity of the blood depending on the content of hemoglobin in the blood and its affinity for oxygen and on the total volume of blood [35]. The high correlation coefficient between hemoglobin concentration and the $VO_{2max}$ value indicates a significant role of this protein in aerobic capacity [71]. A higher level of hemoglobin in the blood in the luteal phase was confirmed by Jurkowski et al. [36]. Increased oxygen availability in tissues during the luteal phase may also result in a higher core temperature during this phase, as well as an elevated level of 2,3-DPG, causing a decrease in the affinity of hemoglobin to oxygen [12, 72]. However, studies carried out by Dombovy et al. [40] showed a slight decrease in the hemoglobin level during the luteal phase. In this research, the differences between phases in the resting level of hemoglobin did not affect the value of $VO_{2max}$, which did not differ between phases.

Stephenson and Kolka [33] found that the resting values of hemoglobin and hematocrit (HCT) are slightly elevated in the luteal phase. Interphase differences in the level of these parameters increased during passive heating and remained unchanged during the exercise with an intensity of approximately 80% $VO_{2max}$. Elevated levels of HCT in the luteal phase were also noted by Stachenfeld et al. [11, 12].

#### *3.1.4. Plasma volume*

Based on the results of earlier studies [33], it may be assumed that higher resting HCT in the luteal phase results from the smaller plasma volume during it. Gaebelein and Senay [32] suggest that the reason for this phenomenon may be an increase in the luteal phase of vascular wall permeability to plasma proteins. Other studies do not support these views [13]. The authors performed an experiment involving seven women, in whom administering a gonadoliberin inhibitor (GnRH) reduced the level of endogenous estradiol and progesterone. Then, successively at intervals of a few days, they added extrinsic preparations containing synthetic derivatives of estradiol and progesterone. In this way, they obtained a ratio of sex hormone concentrations corresponding to, according to the concept of Janse de Jonge [16], the early-follicular, late-follicular, and middle-luteal phases. They found that at elevated levels of both hormones, which correspond to the middle of the luteal phase, the volume of plasma is the largest and constitutes about 17% of the total volume of extracellular fluids. At the same time, in this situation we observe the lowest permeability of blood vessel walls for plasma proteins. Slightly smaller plasma volume and greater permeability of blood vessel walls were observed in a situation corresponding to the late-follicular phase. However, the differences were not statistically significant. Due to the much smaller volume of extracellular fluids, plasma was then 21%. In the situation when only the GnRH inhibitor was administered, the plasma volume was the lowest, and the permeability of blood vessel walls was the largest for albumin. At the same time, the total volume of extracellular fluids was the highest, with a plasma volume of approximately 16%. Differences in the volume of extracellular fluids may be reflected in small changes in the body mass of women during the menstrual cycle [37].

Stephenson and Kolka [33] found that a 9-minute effort at an intensity of about 80% $VO_{2max}$ caused a significantly larger loss of plasma volume during the follicular phase. The percentage changes in plasma volume reached −15.8 and −13.3% in the follicular and luteal phases, respectively [33]. Other authors did not find significant interphase differences in plasma volume changes immediately after exercise and during the restitution period [12, 37, 38, 48].

### 3.2. Anaerobic exercise

In the majority of studies assessing the influence of sex hormones on women's exercise responses, efforts were made of constant submaximal intensity or gradually increasing until reaching maximal oxygen uptake, i.e., "until exhaustion." However, there is little information on the interphase variation in response to typical anaerobic efforts [73–78].

The concept of anaerobic capacity of an organism encompasses a set of factors determining the performance of short-term work, during which large force and maximal generated power are developed. These include skeletal muscle mass, the supply of muscle energy substrates [ATP, phosphocreatine (PCr), glycogen], and enzyme activity of anaerobic processes. The large buffer capacity that allows tolerance of homeostatic disorders and rapid restitution in the pH range is also extremely important [79].

Taking the metabolic effects of estradiol and progesterone into account, it can be assumed that the changing ratio of these hormones during the menstrual cycle effects different physiological responses of women under the influence of anaerobic exercise [80]. The presence of estrogen receptors in the human skeletal muscle [81] and the correlation between strength and high concentrations of 17β-estradiol and progesterone have been found [82]. Furthermore, buffering capacity during the 10-s rowing sprint was greater at a higher concentration of 17β-estradiol [83]. Research suggests that ovarian hormones may influence the rate of PCr resynthesis after eutrophic luteal efforts in eumenorrheic women [84]. Other studies also indicate a faster rate of PCr regeneration after anaerobic efforts in the luteal phase due to the greater work performed in this phase of the menstrual cycle during a series of ten 6-s sprints [85]. This indicates the potential for generating more anaerobic power during the luteal phase of the menstrual cycle (high concentration of 17β-estradiol and progesterone) or just before ovulation (high concentration of 17β-estradiol) compared to the follicular phase. In the literature, however, there is little information on the effect of different levels of hormones on the size of the developed strength or the level of anaerobic power indicators during the menstrual cycle, and their results are not consistent.

While some studies show better results during the luteal phase for single and multiple sprints [85, 86], in others, there were no interphase differences in single or repeated anaerobic cycling tests [87, 88]. Bale and Nelson [89], examining 20 women training swimming, found that they achieved the best results for a distance of 50 m in the follicular phase. Also, Parish and Jakeman [90] found that in comparison with the ovulation period and the luteal phase, the highest maximal and average anaerobic power values were obtained by women in the follicular phase.

However, it should be emphasized that the choice of experiment day in some studies was not hormonally confirmed [86–90]. In many experiments on this subject, the research dates were chosen only by calendar or thermal method. Anovulatory cycles may occur without disturbing the length of the menstrual cycle, while in the case of using the calendar method, this may lead to an erroneous indication of the day of laboratory examination. In turn, a reliable diagnosis of the course of the sexual cycle, based on the measurement of basic body temperature, is possible only after the measurements have been performed in at least three consecutive cycles. The erroneous conclusions concerning the division of the cycle into follicular and luteal phases with the use of the thermal method may additionally be caused by factors such as incorrect method of core temperature measurement, night sleep less than 6 hours, disease states, or the use of hypnotics. Inference based on the results obtained by the authors using the calendar method or thermal method is therefore limited [16].

### *3.2.1. Research based on hormonal verification of menstrual cycle*

The results of research based on hormonal verification of the division of the menstrual cycle into phases indicate lack of significant impact of sex hormones on the values of the developed strength [91] and generated anaerobic power [73]. Nonetheless, other studies [76] show that muscle strength returns to the baseline level faster after strenuous stretch-shortening cycle exercise during the ovulatory phase, when the estrogen level is high, compared with the follicular phase. However, the differences in exercise-induced muscle damage markers (CK, soreness, and low-frequency fatigue) between the two menstrual cycle phases were small.

In the research by Wiecek et al. [75], determining the size of the maximal anaerobic power, a 20-second cycle sprint was used (Wingate test version) [92]. The energy medium of this type of effort regards mainly anaerobic processes consisting in the resynthesis of ATP at the expense of PCr and muscle glycogen. According to the research review, participation of these two processes in ATP synthesis starts from the first seconds of effort, with the participation of the phosphagen energy source in favor of anaerobic glycolysis in subsequent seconds [79]. To obtain fully reliable results, Wiecek et al. [75] performed initial assessment of the correctness and regularity of the menstrual cycle on the basis of the registration of basic body temperature. The correctness of experiment day selection was always verified by hormonal assays. In addition, the studies were repeated in two subsequent menstrual cycles. Each woman performed an anaerobic effort twice in the middle of the follicular phase (days 6–9 of the cycle) and two times in the middle of the luteal phase (5–8 days after ovulation). The first day of menstruation was adopted as the first day of the menstrual cycle. The studies concluded that there are no significant differences in the level of indicators determining anaerobic capacity of women in the follicular and luteal phases of the menstrual cycle. No interphase differences were found in the maximal level or average anaerobic power. The time of obtaining and maintaining maximal power and the rate of decrease in anaerobic power were not different either. The effect of anaerobic metabolism during a 20-second effort at supramaximal intensity is a significant increase in blood lactate concentration, which entails changes in the level of acid-base balance parameters. In both phases of the menstrual cycle, the anaerobic effort caused similar disturbances in the acid-base balance [75].

Also, in the research by Tsampoukos et al. [77], the days for exercise were carefully selected. Eumenorrheic women performed a test comprised of two, 30-s sprints separated by a 2-min break. The test was conducted during the follicular phase, just before ovulation and in the luteal phase. The mutual ovarian hormone system was characterized by adequately low levels of progesterone and 17β-estradiol, low progesterone levels and high levels of 17β-estradiol, and high levels of progesterone and 17β-estradiol. It was found that there are no interphase differences in the maximal level or average anaerobic power. Menstrual cycle hormones also did not affect postexercise changes in metabolic parameters (blood lactate and pH, plasma ammonia) or the rate of regeneration between sprints [77].

Furthermore, during the 6-s cycling sprint, there were no interphase differences in the amount of generated anaerobic power and changes in blood lactate or in the sympatho-adrenergic response tested by the measurement of adrenaline and noradrenaline in the blood [93]. The lack of influence of sex hormones on different exercise responses in the follicular and luteal phases was also demonstrated by studies in which no interphase differences were found in maximal accumulated oxygen deficit and sprint performance in repeated sprint cycling, i.e., three times at 120% $VO_{2max}$ with 20-minute resting periods between consecutive sprints [78]. Also, the 40-yd running time preceded by a 15-minute warm-up (jogging, skipping by moving the legs in various directions, and sprinting alternating with jogging), performed at an ambient temperature of about 32.5°C, did not differ between the early-follicular and middle-luteal phases [94]. Regardless of the menstrual cycle phase, the warm-up triggered an increase in the core temperature of about 1°C, which resulted in a better result during the run [94].

Similar results were also obtained in earlier studies [74]. Domagala et al. [74] obtained results indicating a tendency for smaller increases in lactate concentration and changes in acid-base balance parameters in the luteal phase of the menstrual cycle. In the luteal phase, they also noted a slightly higher rate of lactate concentration restitution after exercise with a supramaximal load; however, the interfacial differences were not statistically significant [74].

However, in the research by Redman and Weatherby [83], in which rowers performed a test of anaerobic power (10-s all-out effort) and capacity (1000-m row), it was found that the peak power output was higher and the 1000-m rowing ergometer time was faster when the concentration of progesterone and estradiol was low (quasi-follicular phase), in contrast to when the levels of both hormones were high (quasi-luteal phase). The concentration of sex hormones was regulated by oral contraceptive pills [83]. Julian et al. [95], by examining female soccer players who performed the Yo-Yo intermittent endurance test, multiple jumps, and 3 × 30 m sprints in the early-follicular phase and in the middle of the luteal phase, showed a reduction in maximal endurance performance during the middle-luteal phase. This effect was not observed for jumping or sprint performance.

### 3.3. Thermoregulation

An important factor conditioning the possibility of performing physical exercise is the efficient functioning of thermoregulation mechanisms. During rest, in thermoneutral conditions, the heat balance of the body is stabilized by the exchange of heat produced in metabolic processes. Heat is exchanged with the environment through conduction and convection, radiation, and evaporation. By these means, approximately 20, 60, and 20%, respectively, of heat is eliminated from the body [96].

During physical exercise, as a result of the intensification of metabolic processes, the thermal balance of the body and the stimulation of thermoregulation systems are disturbed. We observe an increase in the core temperature of the body, depending on the relative load expressed as % $VO_{2max}$, which during efforts at constant intensity is stabilized at an elevated level. The main role in the elimination of excess endogenous heat during physical exercise is played by evaporation of perspiration from the body's surface, constituting about 80% of heat loss [96]. The effectiveness of exercise-based thermoregulation depends on the rate of sweat secretion and external conditions affecting the efficiency of its evaporation, as well as the correct functioning of the circulatory system, on which the heat transfer from the muscles to the surface of the skin depends [96]. After core temperature exceeds the so-called vasodilation threshold, blood flow through the cutaneous vessels steadily increases along with the increase of exercise intensity to about 60–70% $VO_{2max}$, after which it gradually decreases due to the increase in muscular flow [97]. Thermoregulatory reactions also depend on hydration status of the body, the concentration of sodium and calcium ions in body fluids, the degree of acclimation to the conditions under which physical exercise is performed, and the level of physical fitness [96].

The increase in resting body temperature during the luteal phase of the menstrual cycle by about 0.3–0.5°C, as compared to the level during the follicular phase, is the result of the antagonistic effect of progesterone and estradiol on the thermoregulatory system in the hypothalamus [12]. Observations of many authors indicate the relationship between thermoregulatory responses in women and the course of the menstrual cycle [29, 39, 41, 98–100].

#### *3.3.1. Core temperature and sweating*

The average temperature measured in the esophagus ($T_{es}$), in thermoneutral conditions, during a 30-minute exercise at an intensity of 40 and 70% $VO_{2max}$, was higher in the luteal phase [101]. The increase in $T_{es}$ obtained in these studies was the same in both phases of the menstrual cycle [101]. In other studies [102], the temperature measured in the auditory canal ($T_{ty}$), at rest and during exercise tests (60-minute 50% $VO_{2max}$ and during the graded test), was significantly higher in the luteal phase of the menstrual cycle, and $T_{ty}$ increases were slightly higher in follicular phase.

The increases in core temperature, similar in both phases, during submaximal efforts performed in thermoneutral conditions and in conditions of elevated temperature, were also observed in the studies presented by other authors [12, 94, 100, 103]. These results are only partially consistent with the results of this study, during which a higher level of rectal temperature ($T_{re}$) was observed in the luteal phase of the menstrual cycle while performing a 60-minute effort at constant intensity of about 60% $VO_{2max}$ (ambient temperature 22°C) [41]. However, $T_{re}$ increments were comparable in both phases of the menstrual cycle only during the initial minutes of exercise, after which the differences between phases increased due to stabilization of $T_{re}$ in the follicular phase at the level of 38.3°C and its continuous increase to 38.9°C (despite the constant load) in the luteal phase [41].

During a 15-minute exercise at a constant intensity of 70% $VO_{2max}$, performed in an ambient temperature of 18°C, significantly higher $T_{re}$ increments were observed in the follicular phase of the menstrual cycle [39]. In conditions of passive overheating or physical exertion, activation of sweat secretion and dilation of cutaneous blood vessels were observed at higher temperatures as well as a higher intensity of perspiration secretion in the luteal phase [12, 28, 29, 39, 98–102]. There was also later occurrence of perspiration production during exercise tests in the follicular phase [28].

Despite the different course of $T_{re}$ changes in the follicular and luteal phases, the sweat rate was similar in both phases of the menstrual cycle [41]. The authors suggest that this may be related to lower sensitivity of sweat secretion in the luteal phase (sweating rate—increase of core temperature dependency) [41]. However, these results are not confirmed by other laboratory tests, which indicate a slightly higher value in the luteal phase [28, 39, 98] or a similar sensitivity of the perspiration mechanism in both phases [12, 99, 100, 103]. The results obtained during submaximal physical exercise in thermoneutral conditions showed that the increase in rectal temperature in women was lower during the luteal than follicular phase, while the dynamics of sweating were higher in the luteal phase [104].

Tests during which women performed two different stress tests (graded test "to refusal" and 60-minute with 50% intensity of $VO_{2max}$) show that the temperature threshold for starting the perspiration release reaction is higher in the luteal phase and does not depend on the type of exercise [102]. In contrast, the sensitivity of the perspiration production reaction is independent of the menstrual cycle and is higher during the graded test [102]. According to other authors, the effectiveness of perspiration is greater in the luteal phase of the menstrual cycle [104, 105].

Lower core temperature during exercise in the follicular phase may be due to interphase differences in the value of dermal flow and skin temperature. Some studies [39, 98] show that in thermoneutral conditions, at rest and during submaximal efforts, blood flow through the forearm reaches significantly higher values in the luteal phase. The temperature level at which the cutaneous blood vessels dilate, determined on the basis of temperature measurements, $T_{es}$,

$T_{ty}$, and $T_{re}$, shifted toward higher values in the luteal phase by about 0.5°C [39]. However, in other studies, resting blood flow in the forearm did not differ during the menstrual cycle [29]. The exercise-based (30 minutes 80% $VO_{2max}$) increase in cutaneous flow coincided with the increase in core temperature ($T_{es}$) to the level of 37.0°C in the follicular phase and 37.4°C in the luteal phase and stabilized at a significantly higher level during the latter phase [29].

*3.3.2. Skin temperature*

According to some authors, the average skin temperature ($T_{sk}$) is significantly higher in the luteal phase at rest and during submaximal efforts in thermoneutral conditions [100] at the time of heat exposure [99, 103] and during passive overheating [99]. The lack of differences between phases in the $T_{sk}$ values measured at rest as well as during the exercise tests (30 minutes 40% $VO_{2max}$ and 30 minutes 70% $VO_{2max}$) performed in thermoneutral conditions was also demonstrated [101]. Cutaneous flow tended to be higher in the luteal phase, but the resulting interphase differences were not statistically significant [101]. Other studies also showed similar resting values and a comparable course of $T_{sk}$ exercise changes in both phases of the menstrual cycle [12, 41, 106]. Cutaneous flow assumed lower values in the luteal phase [106].

**3.4. Oxidative stress**

The body maintains homeostasis in the scope of redox reactions (prooxidation and antioxidative balance), which affects the proper course of biochemical intracellular processes and intercellular signaling. The condition of redox homeostasis is to maintain balance between the level of reactive oxygen and nitrogen species (RONS) and antioxidant defense. Antioxidative defense is provided by nonenzymatic low-molecular and macromolecular antioxidants and antioxidant enzymes, which together determine total antioxidant capacity. Physical activity gives health benefits by improving, among others, cardiovascular and respiratory system functioning, and metabolic processes as well as by increasing antioxidant capacity [107–109].

*3.4.1. Exercise-based sources of oxygen and nitrogen*

Research has shown that physical exercise influences prooxidation and antioxidative balance [110–114]. The mechanism of RONS formation depends on the duration, intensity of effort, and type of muscle work. An increase in ATP consumption during aerobic efforts results in an increase in the rate of oxidative phosphorylation and, consequently, increased electron leakage in the internal mitochondrial membrane. As a result, amounts larger than at rest of the superoxide anion ($O_2^{\bullet-}$), hydrogen peroxide ($H_2O_2$), and hydroxyl radical ($^{\bullet}OH$), which belong to the reactive oxygen species, are formed [109]. The superoxide anion radical is also formed by the reaction of NADPH oxidase in the sarcoplasmic reticulum and transverse tubules (T-tubules) of the sarcolemma, as well as in the reaction of xanthine oxidase, the activity of which increases after anaerobic efforts [108]. The formation of RONS is promoted by the increase in lactate dehydrogenase activity, lowering the pH value, increasing the concentration of catecholamines, as well as increasing intramuscular temperature [108, 109]. Contractile activity also leads to increased nitric oxide (NO) synthesis by induced nitric oxide synthase (iNOS). The consequence of increased NO synthesis, at a high level of $O_2^{\bullet-}$, is the formation of peroxynitrite ($OONO^-$). Peroxynitrite is a reactive form of nitrogen. Excessive RONS production during exercise can also be the result of myocyte micro-injury associated with activation of the leukocytic system [107, 115].

### 3.4.2. *Markers of oxidative stress*

Oxidative stress is determined by changes in the level of many, various markers (**Table 1**). Different oxidation rates and different antioxidants are evaluated in the research, the changes of which are not always unidirectional [107].

### 3.4.3. *The significance of reactive oxygen and nitrogen species*

The formation of RONS in low concentrations (intracellular signaling) is necessary for the regulation and integration of biochemical processes. They activate primary signaling pathways depending on redox status. The main transcription factor, sensitive to redox status, is the nuclear factor erythroid 2-related factor (Nrf2). Nrf2 activation affects the strengthening of antioxidative defense and cytoprotection. It has been shown that as a result of regular exercise, upregulation of gene expression for peroxisome proliferator-activated receptor-γ coactivator-1α (PGC-1α) occurs, which upregulates Nrf2 in order to regulate the mitochondrial biogenesis. The upstream signals that regulate PGC-1α expression as mitogen-activated protein kinase (MAPK) and nuclear factor κB (NF-κB) are also redox-sensitive. RONS, through

| Markers of oxidative stress | Antioxidants |
|---|---|
| 4-Hydroxynonenal (4-HNE) | Endogenous enzymatic |
| F2-isoprostane | • Superoxide dismutase (SOD) |
| Isoprostanes (8-iso-PGF2α) | • Catalase (CAT) |
| Malondialdehyde (MDA) | • Glutathione peroxidase (GPx) |
| Oxidized low-density lipoprotein (ox-LDL) | • Glutathione reductase (GR) |
| Thiobarbituric acid reactive substance (TBARS) | Endogenous nonenzymatic |
| 8-Hydroxy-2′-deoxyguanosine (8-OHdG) | • Albumin |
| 3-Nitrotyrosine (3-NTR) | • Uric acid |
| Protein carbonyl content (PCC) | • Reduced glutathione (GSH) |
| Advanced oxidation protein products (AOPP) | Exogenous nonenzymatic |
| Oxidized glutathione (GSSG) | • β-Carotene, vitamin E, vitamin C |
| Total oxidative status (TOS) | Total antioxidative capacity (TAC) |
| Oxidative stress index (OSI = TOS/TAC) | |

**Table 1.** Examples of indicators of oxidative stress and antioxidants.

MAPK, activate the NF-κB signaling pathway and, thus, affect the expression of antioxidant enzyme genes such as superoxide dismutase (SOD), catalase (CAT), or glutathione peroxidase (GPx) or glutathione reductase (GR). Therefore, they are responsible for maintaining an appropriate level of endogenous antioxidant defense [107–109, 115].

At high concentrations (oxidative damage level), RONS exhibits inhibitory and damaging effects [107]. Excessive production of RONS with low antioxidant capacity may be the reason for shifting the prooxidation and antioxidant balance toward oxidation and oxidative stress. The consequence of oxidative stress is increased lipid peroxidation, oxidation of thiol groups of proteins, damage to DNA and carbohydrates. Oxidative damage to macromolecules is the cause of disturbance in enzyme activity and permeability of biological membranes [107].

### *3.4.4. Antioxidant effect of estradiol activity*

In women, the antioxidative role is attributed to estrogen. Animal experiments have shown that the amount of $H_2O_2$ formed in the mitochondria of females is lower than in the mitochondria of male rats. The positive effect of estradiol on oxidative stress has also been demonstrated in women. It was found that estradiol reduces the level of reactive oxygen species, and in postmenopausal women, it intensifies oxidative stress, which is counteracted by hormone replacement therapy. Estradiol, acting indirectly through the estrogen receptor, increases antioxidant capacity, affecting activation of the NF-κB signaling pathway, which consequently results in an increase in enzymatic antioxidant capacity [116–119].

### *3.4.5. Redox balance in the menstrual cycle*

An interesting research model was carried out by Massafra et al. [120]. Young women (aged 20–27) participated in the study, declaring a regular menstrual cycle, the length of which ranged from 28 to 30 days. The first day of menstruation was accepted as the first day of the menstrual cycle. Changes in ovarian hormones were monitored based on the daily determinations of 17β-estradiol and progesterone. A preovulatory peak of 17β-estradiol concentration was determined for each woman, which was the "0" point. In relation to the "0" point, three tests were determined in the follicular phase (early, from bleeding to −10; middle, from days −8 to −4; late, from days −2 to 0) and in the luteal phase (early, from days 2 to 4; middle, from days 6 to 10; late, from days 12 to 14). Significant changes in the menstrual cycle were found in erythrocyte GPx activity, with higher values in the period from late follicular to early luteal phases compared to early-follicular phase. This coincided with the elevated level of 17β-estradiol, and the correlation coefficient was 0.8. In this study, there was no effect of 17β-estradiol, progesterone, and LH or FSH on the activity of CAT and SOD in erythrocytes, which were similar throughout the menstrual cycle [120].

In turn, in another study [121] involving 259 regularly menstruating women aged 18–44, it was found that the level of antioxidants in blood serum is dependent on ovarian hormones. Similar appointments for assays were determined as in previous studies [120]. Among others, antioxidant fat-soluble vitamins and carotenoid micronutrients (α-tocopherol, γ-tocopherol, β-carotene, retinol, lutein, lycopene) and ascorbic acid were determined. The concentration of F2-isoprostane was determined as an indicator of lipid oxidation. In most women, the assays were conducted during two menstrual cycles. Among others, it was found that the concentrations of fat-soluble vitamins and ascorbic acid are lower during menstruation. The concentration of fat-soluble vitamins positively correlated with the concentration of 17β-estradiol. The concentration of ascorbic acid also correlated positively with the concentration of 17β-estradiol and progesterone, while it was lower when the concentration of LH was higher. Women with higher ascorbic acid concentrations had lower F2-isoprostane concentrations. In this study, the ratio of $\alpha$- to $\gamma$-tocopherol was associated with an increased risk of anovulatory cycles [121].

While regularly maturing young women (cycle length 26–31 days) were divided into two groups, i.e., ovulating and non-ovulating, it was found that plasma TBARS (lipid oxidation index), whole blood GSH concentration, and CAT, GPX, and GR activity in erythrocytes are similar in both groups in the first (7–9 days) and in the second (22–25 days) mid-menstrual cycle [122]. However, the activity of SOD in erythrocytes, in both measurements, was significantly higher in the non-ovulating group. In ovulating women, there was a significant negative correlation between the concentration of 17β-estradiol in the blood plasma and the activity of SOD in erythrocytes. Research has shown that the lack of ovulation in menstruating women does not affect increased lipid peroxidation. In contrast to previous studies [120], there was no effect of GSH-dependent erythrocyte antioxidant defense, while it was found that lower plasma estradiol resulted in attenuated erythrocyte SOD inhibition and elevated enzyme activity [122].

There are also studies in which it was concluded that women are subjected to oxidative stress for most of the menstrual cycle. In these studies, oxidative stress was assessed on the basis of the reactive oxygen metabolites-derived compound test (d-ROMs), the results of which correspond to the hydroxyperoxide level. The measurement in the blood was performed every 3 days, starting from the first day of menstruation up to the last day of the menstrual cycle (the day before the next menstruation). The level of dROMs was significantly elevated between days 9 and 24 of the menstrual cycle, when there was a peak of 17β-estradiol at low progesterone concentration, as well as when the levels of both hormones were elevated. However, there was no correlation between 17β-estradiol concentration and the level of dROMs; thus, it can be assumed that other factors influenced the increased lipid oxidation [123].

Other studies do not confirm the relationship between oxidative stress and the course of the menstrual cycle. There were no differences in the level of 8-OHdG in the urine (oxidative DNA damage index) between follicular phase, ovulation, and the luteal phase of the menstrual cycle [124]. There were also no differences between TBARS [34, 125] and MDA [125, 126], i.e., lipid oxidation indices, as well as $H_2O_2$ and nitrite/nitrate levels [127], nor in total GSH, GSH, and GSSG concentrations [125]. The effect of hormones during the menstrual cycle on the total activity of SOD and the activity of extracellular superoxide dismutase (EC-SOD) [34] or the total antioxidant capacity were not demonstrated [126]. Also, in older postmenopausal women who did not use hormone replacement therapy, there were no higher levels of dROMs or lower antioxidant capacity compared to premenopausal women of similar age (46–55 years). On the basis of dROM values in both groups of women, the middle oxidative stress level was found, and a slight deficit in antioxidant defense was detected [127]. However, the level of lipid oxidation in older women was higher compared to the young (25–35 years), properly menstruating women who did not use contraceptive pills [127].

It was shown that oral contraception (monophasic pills containing 0.02 mg ethinyl estradiol and 3 mg drospirenone) affects the prooxidative and antioxidant status of young women [128]. Compared to women who do not use oral contraception, they cause a decrease in GSH and glutathione S-transferase (GST), GR, and GPx in the blood while increasing CAT activity and lowering GSSG concentration, resulting in the GSH/GSSG oxidative stress index to not change. These studies show that external modification of the concentration of sex hormones causes catalase to play a main antioxidative role, which confirms the positive correlation between CAT activity and MDA concentration. Increased CAT activity may be the result of accumulation of $H_2O_2$ and other radicals. Detoxification of reactive oxygen species by the GSH system is weakened in this situation [128].

### *3.4.6. Exercise-induced changes in redox balance*

Studies show that high levels of 17β-estradiol in non-training young women with normal biphasic menstrual cycles favor easier elimination of free radicals formed during exercise [34]. Despite the lack of interphase differences in resting TBARS level and SOD activity, after a 30-minute cycling effort with 60% intensity $VO_{2max}$, it was found that the TBARS level decreased in the follicular phase when the 17β-estradiol concentration was higher than during menstruation and the luteal phase. In the luteal phase, however, the activity of SOD in the blood decreased after the effort. Although in none of the phases (menstruation, follicular phase, luteal phase), neither at rest nor after exercise, was there any correlation between the concentration of 17β-estradiol and oxidative stress markers, it was nonetheless found that along with the higher concentration of this hormone, the decrease in SOD activity was lower [34].

In another study [125], in which young women also performed a 30-minute moderate-intensity exercise (about 75–80% $VO_{2max}$) in the follicular and luteal phases of the menstrual cycle, a significant postexercise increase in GSSG concentration was noted during the luteal phase (by 28%), while the concentration of total GSH decreased significantly after exercise only in the follicular phase (by 8%). The concentration of GSH after exercise, regardless of the phase of the menstrual cycle, significantly decreased by about 16–17%. These results show that at higher concentrations of 17β-estradiol (late follicular phase), exercise causes slightly less disturbances of redox homeostasis due to more efficient scavenging free radicals with the participation of glutathione [125].

Amenorrheic and eumenorrheic athletes underwent a 90-minute effort at an intensity of 60% $VO_{2max}$ [129]. The level of 17β-estradiol was significantly lower in amenorrheic women both before and during exercises (30, 60, and 90 minutes) and at 15-minute recovery. In these studies, there was a greater effect of the effort on the oxidative stress markers in amenorrheic women. In this group, at rest and during exercise, GPx activity was higher. Before the effort, GR activity in both groups of women was comparable, but as a result of the effort, it also significantly increased in amenorrheic women. Plasma lipid peroxidation concentration and CAT activity were similar in both groups and did not change in response to physical effort. Contrary to other studies [120], there was a negative correlation between GPx activity and 17β-estradiol concentration, but, simultaneously, GPx activity depended positively on cortisol concentration, which was elevated in the group of amenorrheic women [129].

These results are contrary to those of other researchers [130] who found a positive relationship between GPx activity and estradiol levels both before and after physical exercises. Non-training, young women, during menstruation and the preovulatory phase, performed three isokinetic efforts to exhaustion, consisting of performing maximum alternating concentric and eccentric work of the knee extensor muscles of the dominant lower limb, preceded by a 15-minute submaximal bicycle effort at an intensity of 50% $VO_{2max}$. The concentration of MDA in the blood plasma did not change after exercise, but the activity of SOD and GPx in erythrocytes decreased significantly. The effort-induced changes were lower when the estradiol concentration was higher, what is more, the α-tocopherol supplementation (antioxidant vitamin) did not affect this [130].

Another study [131] showed that a low carbohydrate diet for 3 days (5% carbohydrate, 52% fat, 43% protein), preceded by exertion of glycogen depletion, supports the antioxidant defense system in healthy eumenorrhoeic women, both at rest and during graded exercises performed "until exhaustion," compared to women using a balanced diet at this time (59% carbohydrate, 27% fat, 14% protein). It seems reasonable to assume that the higher daily intake of heme iron, selenium, and α-tocopherol provided with a low carbohydrate diet contributed to the increase of antioxidative capacity by increasing the activity of CAT and increasing the concentration of selenium and α-tocopherol in the plasma, which gave better protection of the cell membranes against peroxidative damage caused by physical effort. This is reflected in the limited release of creatine kinase into the blood, which is an indicator of sarcolemma damage. Physical effort was repeated twice in the follicular phase (6–8 days), when the concentration of 17β-estradiol was low, and twice during the luteal phase (4–6 days after ovulation), when both the concentrations of 17β-estradiol and progesterone in the blood were high. In this study, the phase of the menstrual cycle had only a small effect on antioxidant defenses of blood [131].

### *3.4.7. Sex differences in exercise-induced oxidative stress*

It can be assumed that due to differences in estradiol concentration, disturbances in prooxidative-oxidative balance of the blood after exercise are higher in men than women. In the research carried out by Wiecek et al. [111] among young individuals, it was found that the changes in the prooxidative-antioxidative balance of the blood induced by maximum intensity exercise (graded test) differ in women and in men. In men, there was a significant shift in prooxidant-antioxidant balance toward oxidation without increasing the total plasma antioxidant capacity (TAC). In women, the postexercise changes in total plasma oxidation status (TOS) were low due to the increase in TAC. Exercise-induced changes in TOS concentration depended on $VO_{2max}$ and simultaneously, on the increase in lactate concentration [111]. The lack of such relationships in women may indicate the influence of other factors on postexercise oxidative stress in this group of subjects, such as damage to muscle fibers. Continuing research with the participation of young individuals, it was found that the result of physical effort at maximum intensity is significant, independent of $VO_{2max}$ and $VO_2$ as well as the work intensity (% $VO_{2max}$) at the level of the second ventilatory threshold, increase in concentration of ox-LDL and 3-nitrotyrosin in the blood serum, testifying to similar lipid and protein damage in women and men. The significant increase in TAC after exercise at maximum intensity was the result of micro-damage of muscle fibers that occurred in women [114]. However, when young people performed an anaerobic effort, it was found that with similar disturbances of acid-base balance, changes in TAC, TOS, and oxidative stress index (TOS/TAC) in the blood were the same in both women and men. The changes in concentration of low-molecular nonenzymatic antioxidants induced by this effort were also the same in both sexes. The level of the tested markers was indicative of oxidative stress persisting for at least 24 hours after the end of the work [110]. There was no evidence that anaerobic exercise caused muscle damage [113]. During the first hour after completing anaerobic exercise, there were no changes in the activity of xanthine oxidase (XO) in the blood plasma of men or women. The significant increase in the activity of this enzyme was found 24 hours after the completion of anaerobic exercise. The increase in XO activity in the blood after anaerobic exercise was greater in women than men. At the same time, the postexercise increase in XO activity was negatively correlated with the amount of total work performed during anaerobic exercise and with mean and peak anaerobic power, which were significantly lower in women [113]. In turn, the 45-minute submaximal (50% $VO_{2max}$) effort ending with a 15-minute eccentric exercise [downhill run (−4.5°)] caused oxidative damage to lipids only in women [112]. An increase in ox-LDL concentration indicated redox balance disturbances. In men, regardless of the type of muscle work (eccentric, concentric), submaximal running efforts did not cause oxidative stress. The probable cause of these gender differences was the higher antioxidant capacity of men's blood dependent on greater physical performance [112]. In the above studies, however, the phase of the menstrual cycle was not taken into account; women performed the exercise either during the follicular phase or in a randomly selected phase. Nonetheless, the results indicate that changes in redox balance among women depend on the intensity of the effort and on the type of muscle work involved.

## 4. Conclusion

Despite many years of interest in this subject, the current research does not allow to draw unambiguous conclusions about the impact of the changing level of sex hormones during individual phases of the menstrual cycle on the exercise capacity of women. There are indications that in the luteal phase, the capacity to perform efforts based mainly on aerobic energy transformations does increase. For example, in one of recent studies [132], an increase in cardiac and respiratory efficiency in the luteal phase of the menstrual cycle for normal-weight females was found, where as in overweight and obese individuals, there was an overall decrease in fitness capacity along with an increase in body mass index (BMI). However, the differences between groups noted by one researcher in the measured effects of the applied test are not confirmed by observations of other authors [133]. Often, however, differences in the results obtained by women in the pre- and postovulatory phase are small. According to a review of studies on women's exercise capacity, in most experiments, efforts were applied with constant submaximal intensity or gradually increasing until the oxygen uptake was achieved. However, there is little information on intergroup variation in response to typical anaerobic efforts. These studies, as one of the most recent [134], indicate a lack of hormone influence in the menstrual cycle on anaerobic efficiency indices. But these tests also provide divergent results.

The question arises as to why there are still no studies that explicitly determine the exercise capacity of women depending on the phase of the menstrual cycle [135].

Difficulties in undertaking research on exercise-related reactions in women lie, inter alia, in obtaining volunteers for research, especially those non-training ones if the experiment requires the implementation of very high intensity efforts. No physical examinations involve large groups of women. Usually, the research group consists of several to a dozen people. The problem is also obtaining the right motivation of the studied women to fully carry out their potential capabilities during laboratory exercise tests. The reason for the discrepancy of some results may be the determination of test date based on measurements of basic body temperature without hormonal determinations. On the other hand, the source of often conflicting results, given by different authors using sex hormone markers, may be the terminology used to determine the location of the performed laboratory test in the course of the menstrual cycle. Some authors use the division of menstrual cycle into follicular and luteal phases, without specifying the days on which the tests were performed and/or concentrations of estradiol and progesterone determined. Considering the changing ratio of these hormones during the menstrual cycle, the following division seems to be more appropriate: early-follicular (low estradiol and progesterone), late-follicular (elevated estradiol and low progesterone), and middle-luteal (high estradiol and progesterone levels) [16] or to reference the day of testing to the day of ovulation [120]. Difficulties in comparing the results obtained by different authors also result from significant differences in the age and level of physical activity of the surveyed women, or from the variety of applied stress tests and performed assays, which mainly concern markers of oxidative stress. Different methodological approaches and inconsistent presentation of data are a limitation when comparing the results of women obtained by them depending on the changing hormone concentrations of the menstrual cycle. So far, it has not been specified whether it is necessary to take the phase of the menstrual cycle into account in sports diagnostics, e.g., during stress tests that check the physical performance of women training different sports. Also, comparisons between exercise reactions of men and women may be imprecise due to methodological differences. A comprehensive and multi-aspect study of the exercise should be carried out, involving training and non-training women of all ages, in the pre- and postmenopausal period, as well as those using and not using hormonal contraceptives or hormone replacement therapy, which would precisely characterize whether there are differences in biochemical-physiological adaptation to the efforts of varying intensity and type of work and the course of changes in the recovery period, related to the level of hormones in the menstrual cycle.

## Acknowledgements

This work was supported by the Faculty of Physical Education and Sports, University of Physical Education in Krakow, (Poland) under Grant 153/BS/INB/2018.

## Conflict of interest

No conflict of interest was reported.

## Author details

Magdalena Wiecek

Address all correspondence to: magdalena.wiecek@awf.krakow.pl

Department of Physiology and Biochemistry, Faculty of Physical Education and Sport, University of Physical Education, Krakow, Poland

## References

[1] Roupas ND, Georgopoulos NA. Menstrual function in sports. Hormones. 2011;**10**(2): 104-116. DOI: 10.14310/horm.2002.1300

[2] Fischetto G, Sax A. The menstrual cycle and performance. New Studies in Athletics. 2013;**3/4**:57-69

[3] Arena B, Maffulli N, Maffulli F, Morelo MA. Reproductive hormones and menstrual changes with exercise in female athletes. Sports Medicine. 1995;**19**(4):278-287. DOI: 10.2165/00007256-199519040-00005

[4] De Souza MJ. Menstrual disturbances in athletes: A focus on luteal phase defects. Medicine and Science in Sports and Exercise. 2003;**35**(9):1553-1563. DOI: 10.1249/01.MSS.0000084530.31478.DF

[5] Bale P. Body composition and menstrual irregularities of female athletes. Are they precursors of anorexia? Sports Medicine. 1994;**17**(6):347-352. DOI: 10.2165/00007256-199417060-00001

[6] Gibbs JC, Nattiv A, Barrack MT, Williams NI, Rauh MJ, Nichols JF, De Souza MJ. Low bone density risk is higher in exercising women with multiple triad risk factors. Medicine and Science in Sports and Exercise. 2014;**46**(1):167-176. DOI: 10.1249/MSS.0b013e3182a03b8b

[7] De Souza MJ, Koltun KJ, Etter CV, Southmayd EA. Current status of the female athlete triad: Update and future directions. Current Osteoporosis Reports. 2017;**15**(6):577-587. DOI: 10.1007/s11914-017-0412-x

[8] Mehta J, Thompson B, Kling JM. The female athlete triad: It takes a team. Cleveland Clinic Journal of Medicine. **85**(4):313-320. DOI: 10.3949/ccjm.85a.16137

[9] Ashley CD, Kramer ML, Bishop P. Estrogen and substrate metabolism. Sports Medicine. 2000;**29**(4):221-227. DOI: 10.2165/00007256-200029040-00001

[10] Lebrun CM, Rumball JS. Relationship between athletic performance and menstrual cycle. Current Women's Health Reports. 2001;**1**(3):232-240

[11] Stachenfeld NS, DiPietro L, Kokoszka CA, Silva C, Keefe DL, Nadel ER. Physiological variability of fluid-regulation hormones in young women. Journal of Applied Physiology. 1999;**86**:1092-1096. DOI: 10.1152/jappl.1999.86.3.1092

[12] Stachenfeld NS, Celso S, Keefe DL. Estrogen modifies the temperature effects of progesterone. Journal of Applied Physiology. 2000;**88**:1643-1649. DOI: 10.1152/jappl.2000.88.5.1643

[13] Stachenfeld NS, Taylor HS. Effects of estrogen and progesterone administration on extracellular fluid. Journal of Applied Physiology. 2004;**96**(3):101-108. DOI: 10.1152/japplphysiol.01032.2003

[14] Hatta H, Atomi Y, Shinohara S, Yamamoto Y, Yamada S. The effects of ovarian hormones on glucose and fatty acid oxidation during exercise in female ovariectomized rats. Hormone and Metabolic Research. 1988;**20**(10):609-611. DOI: 10.1055/s-2007-1010897

[15] Kendrick ZV, Steffen CA, Rumsey WL, Goldberg DI. Effect of estradiol on tissue glycogen metabolism in exercised oophorectomized rats. Journal of Applied Physiology. 1987;**63**:492-496. DOI: 10.1152/jappl.1987.63.2.492

[16] Janse de Jonge XA. Effects of the menstrual cycle on exercise performance. Sports Medicine. 2003;**33**(11):833-851. DOI: 10.2165/00007256-200333110-00004

[17] Nicklas BJ, Hackney AC, Sharp RL. The menstrual cycle and exercise: Performance, muscle glycogen, and substrate responses. International Journal of Sports Medicine. 1989;**10**(4):264-269. DOI: 10.1055/s-2007-1024913

[18] Bunt JC. Metabolic actions of estradiol: Significance for acute and chronic exercise responses. Medicine and Science in Sports and Exercise. 1990;**22**(3):286-290. DOI: 10.1249/00005768-199006000-00003

[19] Hackney AC. Effects of the menstrual cycle on resting muscle glycogen. Hormone and Metabolic Research. 1991;**22**(12):647. DOI: 10.1055/s-2007-1004994

[20] Hackney AC, McCracken-Compton M, Ainsworth B. Substrate metabolism responses to submaximal exercise in the mid-follicular and mid-luteal phases of the menstrual cycle. International Journal of Sport Nutrition. 1994;**4**(3):299-308

[21] Hornum M, Cooper DM, Brasel JA, Bueno A, Sietsema KE. Exercise-induced changes in circulating growth factors with cyclic variation in plasma estradiol in women. Journal of Applied Physiology. 1997;**82**(6):1946-1951. DOI: 10.1152/jappl.1997.82.6.1946

[22] D'Eon TM, Sharoff C, Chipkin SR, Grow D, Ruby BC, Braun B. Regulation of exercise carbohydrate metabolism by estrogen and progesterone in women. American Journal of Physiology, Endocrinology and Metabolism. 2002;**283**(5):E1046-E1055. DOI: 10.1152/ajpendo.00271.2002

[23] Hansen FM, Fahmy N, Nielsen JH. The influence of sexual hormones on lypogenesis and lipolysis in rat fat cells. Acta Endocrinologica. 1980;**95**:566-570. DOI: 10.1530/acta.0.0950566

[24] Hansen AP, Wecke J. Fasting serum growth hormone levels and GH responses to exercise during normal menstrual cycles and cycles of oral contraceptives. Scandinavian Journal of Clinical and Laboratory Investigation. 1974;**34**:199-205. DOI: 10.3109/00365517409081707

[25] Isacco L, Boisseau N. Sex hormones and substrate metabolism during endurance exercise. In: Hackney AC, editor. Sex Hormones, Exercise and Women. Scientific and Clinical Aspects. 1st ed. Basel: Springer International Publishing; 2017. pp. 35-58. DOI: 10.1007/978-3-319-44558-8

[26] Bayliss DA, Millhorn DE. Central neural mechanisms of progesterone action: Application to the respiratory system. Journal of Applied Physiology. 1992;**73**:393-404. DOI: 10.1152/jappl.1992.73.2.393

[27] Das TK, Jana H. Basal oxygen consumption during different phases of menstrual cycle. Indian Journal of Medical Research. 1991;**94**:16-19

[28] Grucza R, Pekkarinen H, Titov EK, Kononoff A, Hänninen O. Influence of the menstrual cycle and oral contraceptives on thermoregulatory responses to exercise in young women. European Journal of Applied Physiology. 1993;**67**:279-285

[29] Kolka MA, Stephenson LA. Effect of luteal phase elevation in core temperature on forearm blood flow during exercise. Journal of Applied Physiology. 1997;**82**(4):1079-1083. DOI: 10.1152/jappl.1997.82.4.1079

[30] Charkoudian N, Johnson JM. Female reproductive hormones and thermoregulatory control of skin blood flow. Exercise and Sport Sciences Reviews. 2000;**28**(3):108-112

[31] Fortney SM, Beckett WS, Carpenter AJ, Davis J, Drew H, LaFrance ND, Rock JA, Tankersley CG, Vroman NB. Changes in plasma volume during bed rest: Effects of menstrual cycle and estrogen administration. Journal of Applied Physiology. 1988;**65**(2):525-533. DOI: 10.1152/jappl.1988.65.2.525

[32] Gaebelein CJ, Senay L. Vascular volume dynamics during ergometer exercise at different menstrual phases. European Journal of Applied Physiology. 1982;**50**:1-11. DOI: 10.1007/BF00952239

[33] Stephenson LA, Kolka MA. Plasma volume during heat stress and exercise in women. European Journal of Applied Physiology. 1988;**57**:373-381. DOI: 10.1007/BF00417979

[34] Joo MH, Maehata E, Adachi T, Ishida A, Murai F, Mesaki N. The relationship between exercise-induced oxidative stress and the menstrual cycle. European Journal of Applied Physiology. 2004;**93**(1-2):82-86. DOI: 10.1007/s00421-004-1168-4

[35] Bassett DR, Howley ET. Limiting factors for maximum oxygen uptake and determinants of endurance performance. Medicine and Science in Sports and Exercise. 2000;**32**:70-84. DOI: 10.1097/00005768-200001000-00012

[36] Jurkowski JE, Jones NL, Toews CJ, Sutton JR. Effects of the menstrual cycle on blood lactate, $O_2$ delivery, and performance during exercise. Journal of Applied Physiology. 1981;**51**(6):1493-1499. DOI: 10.1152/jappl.1981.51.6.1493

[37] Bemben DA, Salm PC, Salm AJ. Ventilatory and blood lactate responses to maximal treadmill exercise during the menstrual cycle. Journal of Sports Medicine and Physical Fitness. 1995;**35**(4):257-262

[38] McCracken M, Ainsworth B, Hackney AC. Effects of the menstrual cycle phase on the blood lactate responses to exercise. European Journal of Applied Physiology. 1994;**69**:174-175. DOI: 10.1007/BF00609412

[39] Hessemer V, Bruck K. Influence of menstrual cycle on thermoregulatory, metabolic, and heart rate responses to exercise at night. Journal of Applied Physiology. 1985;**59**(6):1911-1917. DOI: 10.1152/jappl.1985.59.6.1911

[40] Dombovy ML, Bonekat HW, Williams TJ, Staats BA. Exercise performance and ventilatory response in the menstrual cycle. Medicine and Science in Sports and Exercise. 1987;**19**(2):111-117. DOI: 10.1249/00005768-198704000-00008

[41] Pivarnik JM, Marichal CJ, Spillman T, Morrow JR. Menstrual cycle phase affects temperature regulation during endurance exercise. Journal of Applied Physiology. 1992;**72**(2):543-548. DOI: 10.1152/jappl.1992.72.2.543

[42] Galliven EA, Singh A, Michelson D, Bina S, Gold PW, Deuster PA. Hormonal and metabolic responses to exercise across time of day and menstrual cycle phase. Journal of Applied Physiology. 1997;**83**(6):1822-1831. DOI: 10.1152/jappl.1997.83.6.1822

[43] Dean TM, Perreault L, Mazzeo RS, Horton TJ. No effect of menstrual cycle phase on lactate threshold. Journal of Applied Physiology. 2003;**95**:2537-2543. DOI: 10.1152/japplphysiol.00672.2003

[44] Zielinski P, Cempla J, Klimek AT, Domagala M. The effect of menstruation on chosen physiological and biochemical reactions caused by the physical effort with the submaximal intensity. Biology of Sport. 2003;**20**(1):53-67

[45] Redman LM, Scroop GC, Norman RJ. Impact of menstrual cycle phase on the exercise status of young, sedentary women. European Journal of Applied Physiology. 2003;**90**(5-6):505-513. DOI: 10.1007/s00421-003-0889-0

[46] Schoene RB, Robertson HT, Pierson DJ, Peterson AP. Respiratory drives and exercise in menstrual cycles of athletic and nonathletic women. Journal of Applied Physiology. 1981;**50**:1300-1305. DOI: 10.1152/jappl.1981.50.6.1300

[47] Das TK. Effects of the menstrual cycle on timing and depth of breathing at rest. Indian Journal of Physiology and Pharmacology. 1998;**42**(4):498-502

[48] De Souza MJ, Maguire MS, Rubin KR, Maresh CM. Effects of menstrual phase and amenorrhea on exercise performance in runners. Medicine and Science in Sports and Exercise. 1990;**22**(5):575-580. DOI: 10.1249/00005768-199010000-00006

[49] Moran VH, Leathard HL, Coley J. Cardiovascular functioning during the menstrual cycle. Clinical Physiology. 2000;**20**(6):496-504. DOI: 10.1046/j.1365-2281.2000.00285.x

[50] Reinhard U, Muller PH, Schmulling RM. Determination of anaerobic threshold by the ventilation equivalent in normal individuals. Respiration. 1979;**38**(1):36-42. DOI: 10.1159/000194056

[51] Skinner JS, McLellan TH. The transition from aerobic to anaerobic metabolism. Research Quarterly for Exercise and Sport. 1980;**51**(1):234-248. DOI: 10.1080/02701367.1980.10609285

[52] Wasserman K, Beaver WL, Whipp BJ. Mechanisms and patterns of blood lactate increase during exercise in man. Medicine and Science in Sports and Exercise. 1986;**18**(3):344-352. DOI: 10.1249/00005768-198606000-00017

[53] Binder RK, Wonisch M, Corra U, Cohen-Solal A, Vanhees L, Saner H, Schmid J-P. Methodological approach to the first and second lactate threshold in incremental cardiopulmonary exercise testing. European Journal of Cardiovascular Prevention and Rehabilitation. 2008;**15**(6):726-734. DOI: 10.1097/HJR.0b013e328304fed4

[54] Faude O, Kindermann W, Meyer T. Lactate threshold concepts. How valid are they? Sports Medicine. 2009;**39**:469-490. DOI: 0112-1642/09/0006-0469/$49.95/0

[55] Beaver WL, Wasserman K, Whipp BJ. A new method for detecting anaerobic threshold by gas exchange. Journal of Applied Physiology. 1986;**60**:2020-2027. DOI: 10.1152/jappl.1986.60.6.2020

[56] Meyer T, Faude O, Scharhag J, Urhausen A, Kindermann W. Is lactic acidosis a cause of exercise induced hyperventilation at the respiratory compensation point? British Journal of Sports Medicine. 2004;**38**:622-625. DOI: 10.1136/bjsm.2003.007815

[57] Lamont LS. Lack of influence of the menstrual cycle on blood lactate. The Physician and Sports Medicine. 1986;**14**(11):159-163. DOI: 10.1080/00913847.1986.11709230

[58] Preston RJ, Aaron P, Heenan P, Wolfe LA. Physicochemical analysis of phasic menstrual cycle effects on acid-base balance. American Journal of Physiology Regulatory, Integrative and Comparative Physiology. 2001;**80**:R481-R487. DOI: 10.1152/ajpregu.2001.280.2.R481

[59] Lavoie JM, Dionne N, Helie R, Brisson GR. Menstrual cycle phase dissociation of blood glucose homeostasis during exercise. Journal of Applied Physiology. 1987;**62**(3):1084-1089. DOI: 10.1152/jappl.1987.62.3.1084

[60] Devries MC, Hamadeh MJ, Phillips SM, Tarnopolsky MA. Menstrual cycle phase and sex influence muscle glycogen utilization and glucose turnover during moderate-intensity endurance exercise. American Journal of Physiology. Regulatory, Integrative and Comparative Physiology. 2006;**291**(4):R1120-R1128. DOI: 10.1152/ajpregu.00700.2005

[61] Campbell SE, Angus DJ, Febbraio MA. Glucose kinetics and exercise performance during phases of the menstrual cycle: Effect of glucose ingestion. American Journal of Physiology. Endocrinology and Metabolism. 2001;**281**:E817-E825. DOI: 10.1152/ajpendo.2001.281.4.E817

[62] Hackney AC. Influence of oestrogen on muscle glycogen utilization during exercise. Acta Physiologica Scandinavica. 1999;**167**:273-274. DOI: 10.1046/j.1365-201x.1999.00605.x

[63] Zderic TW, Coggan AR, Fuby BC. Glucose kinetics and substrate oxidation during exercise in the follicular and luteal phases. Journal of Applied Physiology. 2001;**90**:447-453. DOI: 10.1097/00005768-199805001-01469

[64] Wenz M, Berend JZ, Lynch NA, Chappell S, Hackney AC. Substrate oxidation at rest and during exercise: Effects of menstrual cycle phase and diet composition. Journal of Physiology and Pharmacology. 1997;**48**:851-860

[65] Suh SH, Casazza GA, Horning MA, Miller BF, Brooks GA. Luteal and follicular glucose fluxes during rest and exercise in 3-h postabsorptive women. Journal of Applied Physiology. 2002;**93**:42-50. DOI: 10.1152/japplphysiol.01080.2001

[66] Horton TJ, Miller EK, Glueck D, Tench K. No effect of menstrual cycle phase on glucose kinetics and fuel oxidation during moderate-intensity exercise. American Journal of Physiology, Endocrinology and Metabolism. 2002;**282**:E752-E762. DOI: 10.1152/ajpendo.00238.2001

[67] Bailey SP, Zacher CM, Mittleman KD. Effect of menstrual cycle phase on carbohydrate supplementation during prolonged exercise to fatigue. Journal of Applied Physiology. 2000;**88**(2):690-697. DOI: 10.1152/jappl.2000.88.2.690

[68] Vaiksaar S, Jurimae J, Maestu J, Purge P, Kalytka S, Shakhlina L, Jurimae T. No effect of menstrual cycle phase and oral contraceptive use on endurance performance in rowers. The Journal of Strength and Conditioning Research. 2011;**25**(6):1571-1578. DOI: 10.1519/JSC.0b013e3181df7fd2

[69] Vaiksaar S, Jurimae J, Maestu J, Purge P, Kalytka S, Shakhlina L, Jurimae T. No effect of menstrual cycle phase on fuel oxidation during exercise in rowers. European Journal of Applied Physiology. 2011;**111**(6):1027-1034. DOI: 10.1007/s00421-010-1730-1

[70] Smekal G, von Duvillard SP, Frigo P, Tegelhofer T, Pokan R, Hofmann P, Tschan H, Baron R, Wonisch M, Renezeder K, Bachl N. Menstrual cycle: No effect on exercise cardiorespiratory variables or blood lactate concentration. Medicine and Science in Sports and Exercise. 2007;**39**(7):1098-1106. DOI: 10.1249/mss.0b013e31805371e7

[71] Green HJ, Carter S, Grant S, Tupling R, Coates G, Ali M. Vascular volumes and hematology in male and female runners and cyclists. European Journal of Applied Physiology. 1999;**79**:244-250. DOI: 10.1007/s004210050502

[72] Denis P, Cazor JL, Feret J, Weisang E. Lefrancois. 2,3-Diphosphoglycerate red cell concentration changes during the menstrual cycle in women. Biomedicine. 1976;**25**(4):144-147

[73] Giacomoni M, Bernard T, Gavarry O, Altare S, Falgairette G. Influence of the menstrual cycle phase and menstrual symptoms on maximal anaerobic performance. Medicine and Science in Sports and Exercise. 2000;**32**(2):486-492. DOI: 10.1097/00005768-200002000-00034

[74] Domagala M, Cempla J, Bawelski M, Zielinski P. Changes in a lactate, $H^+$ ions and base excess concentrations during exercises of different intensities in relation to the phase of menstrual cycle. Biology of Sport. 2001;**18**(4):311-319

[75] Wiecek M, Szymura J, Maciejczyk M, Cempla J, Szygula Z. Effect of sex and menstrual cycle in women on starting speed, anaerobic endurance and muscle power. Physiology International. 2016;**103**(1):127-132. DOI: 10.1556/036.103.2016.1.13

[76] Sipaviciene S, Daniuseviciute L, Kliziene I, Kamandulis S, Skurvydas A. Effects of estrogen fluctuation during the menstrual cycle on the response to stretch-shortening exercise in females. BioMed Research International. 2013;**2013**:243572. DOI: 10.1155/2013/243572

[77] Tsampoukos A, Peckham EA, James R, Nevill ME. Effect of menstrual cycle phase on sprinting performance. European Journal of Applied Physiology. 2010;**109**(4):659-667. DOI: 10.1007/s00421-010-1384-z

[78] Shaharudin S, Ghosh AK, Ismail AA. Anaerobic capacity of physically active eumenorrheic females at mid-luteal and mid-follicular phases of ovarian cycle. Journal of Sports Medicine and Physical Fitness. 2011;**51**(4):576-582

[79] Morales-Alamo D, Calbet JAL. Free radicals and sprint exercise in humans. Free Radical Research. 2014;**48**(1):30-42. DOI: 10.3109/10715762.2013.825043

[80] Oosthuyse T, Bosch AN. The effect of the menstrual cycle on exercise metabolism. Implications for exercise performance in Eumenorrhoeic women. Sports Medicine. 2010;**40**(3):207-227. DOI: 0112-1642/10/0003-0207/$49.95/0

[81] Lemoine S, Granier P, Tiffoche C, Rannou-Bekono F, Thieulant ML, Delamarche P. Estrogen receptor alpha mRNA in human skeletal muscles. Medicine and Science in Sports and Exercise. 2003;**35**(3):439-443. DOI: 10.1249/01.MSS.0000053654.14410.78

[82] Taaffe DR, Newman AB, Haggerty CL, Colbert LH, de Rekeneire N, Visser M, Goodpaster BH, Nevitt MC, Tylavsky FA, Harris TB. Estrogen replacement, muscle composition, and physical function: The health ABC study. Medicine and Science in Sports and Exercise. 2005;**37**(10):1741-1747. DOI: 10.1249/01.mss.0000181678.28092.31

[83] Redman LM, Weatherby RP. Measuring performance during menstrual cycle: A model using oral contraceptives. Medicine and Science in Sports and Exercise. 2004;**36**(1):130-136. DOI: 10.1249/01.MSS.0000106181.52102.99

[84] Harber VJ, Petersen SR, Chilibeck PD. Thyroid hormone concentrations and muscle metabolism in amenorrheic and eumenorrheic athletes. Canadian Journal of Applied Physiology. 1998;**23**:293-306. DOI: 10.1139/h98-017

[85] Middleton LE, Wenger HA. Effects of menstrual phase on performance and recovery in intense intermittent activity. European Journal of Applied Physiology. 2006;**96**(1):53-58. DOI: 10.1007/s00421-005-0073-9

[86] Masterson G. The impact of menstrual cycle phases on anaerobic power performance in collegiate women. Journal of Strength and Conditioning Research. 1999;**13**:325-329

[87] Bushman B, Masterson G, Nelsen J. Anaerobic power performance and the menstrual cycle: Eumenorrheic and oral contraceptive users. Journal of Sports Medicine and Physical Fitness. 2006;**46**(1):132-137

[88] Miskec CM, Potteiger JA, Nau KL, Zebas CJ. Do varying environment and menstrual cycle conditions affect anaerobic power output in female athletes. Journal of Strength and Conditioning Research. 1997;**11**:219-223. DOI: 10.1519/1533-4287(1997)011<0219:DVEAMC>2.3.CO;2

[89] Bale P, Nelson G. The effects of menstruation on performance of swimmers. Australian Journal of Science and Medicine in Sport. 1985;**3**:19-22

[90] Parish H, Jakeman PM. The effects of menstruation upon repeated maximal sprint performance. Journal of Sports Sciences. 1987;**1**:78

[91] Friden C, Hirschberg AL, Saartok T. Muscle strength and endurance do not significantly vary across 3 phases of the menstrual cycle in moderately active premenopausal women. Clinical Journal of Sport Medicine. 2003;**13**(4):238-241. DOI: 10.1097/00042752-200307000-00007

[92] Inbar O, Bar-Or O, Skinner JS. Characteristics of the Wingate anaerobic test: Relative aerobic and anaerobic contributions. In: Inbar O, Bar-Or O, Skinner JS, editors. The Wingate Anaerobic Test. Champaign: Human Kinetics; 1996. pp. 35-37

[93] Botcazou M, Gratas-Delamarche A, Allain S, Jacob C, Bentué-Ferrer D, Delamarche P, Zouhal H. Influence of menstrual cycle phase on catecholamine response to sprint exercise in the woman. Applied Physiology Nutrition and Metabolism. 2006;**31**(5):604-611. DOI: 10.1139/h06-038

[94] Somboonwong J, Chutimakul L, Sanguanrungsirikul S. Core temperature changes and sprint performance of elite female soccer players after a 15-minute warm-up in hot-humid environment. Journal of Strength and Conditioning Research. 2015;**29**(1):262-269. DOI: 10.1519/JSC.0b013e3182aa5f2f

[95] Julian R, Hecksteden A, Fullagar HH, Meyer T. The effects of menstrual cycle phase on physical performance in female soccer players. PLoS One. 2017;**12**(3):e0173951. DOI: 10.1371/journal.pone.0173951

[96] Kenney WL, Wilmore JH, Costill DL. Exercise in hot and cold environments. In: Kenney WL, Wilmore JH, Costill DL, editors. Physiology of Sport and Exercise. 5th ed. Champaign: Human Kinetics; 2011. pp. 283-307

[97] Smolander J, Kolari P, Korhonen O, Ilmarinen R. Skin blood flow during incremental exercise in thermoneutral and hot dry environment. European Journal of Applied Physiology and Occupational Physiology. 1987;**56**(3):273-280. DOI: 10.1007/BF00690892

[98] Hessemer V, Bruck K. Influence of menstrual cycle on shivering, skin blood flow, and sweating responses measured at night. Journal of Applied Physiology. 1985;**59**(6):1902-1910. DOI: 10.1152/jappl.1985.59.6.1902

[99] Kolka MA, Stephenson LA. Control of sweating during the human menstrual cycle. European Journal of Applied Physiology. 1989;**58**:890-895. DOI: 10.1007/BF02332224

[100] Fukuoka Y, Kaneko Y, Takita C, Hirakawa M, Kagawa H, Nakamura Y. The effects of exercise intensity on thermoregulatory responses to exercise in women. Physiology and Behavior. 2002;**76**:567-574. DOI: 10.1016/S0031-9384(02)00781-3

[101] Hirata K, Nagasaka T, Hirai A, Hirashita M, Takahata T, Nunomura T. Effects of human menstrual cycle on thermoregulatory vasodilation during exercise. European Journal of Applied Physiology. 1986;**54**:559-565. DOI: 10.1007/BF00943341

[102] Pokora I, Grucza R. Thermoregulatory responses to exercise in women during follicular and luteal phase of the menstrual cycle. Biology of Sport. 2000;**17**(1):13-24

[103] Carpenter AJ, Nunneley SA. Endogenous hormones subtly alter women's response to heat stress. Journal of Applied Physiology. 1988;**65**(5):2313-2317. DOI: 10.1152/jappl.1988.65.5.2313

[104] Kaciuba-Uscilko H, Grucza R. Gender differences in thermoregulation. Current Opinion in Clinical Nutrition and Metabolic Care. 2001;**4**:533-536

[105] Garcia AMC, Lacerda MG, Fonseca IAT, Reis FM, Rodrigues LOC, Silami-Garcia E. Luteal phase of the menstrual cycle increases sweating rate during exercise. Brazilian Journal of Medical and Biological Research. 2006;**39**:1255-1261. DOI: 10.1590/S0100-879X2006000900014

[106] Frascarolo P, Schutz Y, Jequier E. Decreased thermal conductance during the luteal phase of the menstrual cycle in women. Journal of Applied Physiology. 1990;**69**:2029-2033

[107] Durackova Z. Some current insights into oxidative stress. Physiological Research. 2010;**59**:459-469

[108] Powers SK, Talbert EE, Adhihetty PJ. Reactive oxygen and nitrogen species as intracellular signals in skeletal muscle. The Journal of Physiology. 2011;**9**:2129-2138. DOI: 10.1113/jphysiol.2010.201327

[109] He F, Li J, Liu Z, Chuang CC, Yang W, Zuo L. Redox mechanism of reactive oxygen species in exercise. Frontiers in Physiology. 2016;**7**:486. DOI: 10.3389/fphys.2016.00486

[110] Wiecek M, Maciejczyk M, Szymura J, Szygula Z, Kantorowicz M. Changes in non-enzymatic antioxidants in the blood following anaerobic exercise in men and women. PLoS One. 2015;**10**(11):e0143499. DOI: 10.1371/journal.pone.0143499

[111] Wiecek M, Maciejczyk M, Szymura J, Szygula Z. Changes in oxidative stress and acid-base balance in men and women following maximal-intensity physical exercise. Physiological Research. 2015;**64**(1):93-102

[112] Wiecek M, Maciejczyk M, Szymura J, Szygula Z. Sex differences in oxidative stress after eccentric and concentric exercise. Redox Report. 2017;**22**(6):478-485. DOI: 10.1080/13510002.2017.1304195

[113] Wiecek M, Maciejczyk M, Szymura J, Kantorowicz M, Szygula Z. Impact of single anaerobic exercise on delayed activation of endothelial xanthine oxidase in men and women. Redox Report. 2017;**22**(6):367-376. DOI: 10.1080/13510002.2016.1238991

[114] Wiecek M, Maciejczyk M, Szymura J, Szygula Z. Effect of maximal-intensity exercise on systemic nitro-oxidative stress in men and women. Redox Report. 2017;**22**(4):176-182. DOI: 10.1080/13510002.2016.1169622

[115] Nikolaidis MG, Kyparos A, Spanou C, Paschalis V, Theodorou AA, Vrabas IS. Redox biology of exercise: An integrative and comparative consideration of some overlooked issues. The Journal of Experimental Biology. 2012;**215**:1615-1625. DOI: 10.1242/jeb.067470

[116] Ayers S, Abplanalp W, Liu JH, Subbiah TR. Mechanism involved in the protective effect of estradiol-17β on lipid peroxidation and DNA damage. American Journal of Physiology. 1998;**274**:E1002-E1008. DOI: 10.1152/ajpendo.1998.274.6.E1002

[117] Tiidus PM. Estrogen and gender effects on muscle damage, inflammation, and oxidative stress. Canadian Journal of Applied Physiology. 2000;**25**(4):274-287. DOI: 10.1139/h00-022

[118] Vina J, Gambini J, Lopez-Grueso R, Abdelaziz KM, Jove M, Borras C. Females live longer than males: Role of oxidative stress. Current Pharmaceutical Design. 2011;**17**:3959-3965. DOI: 10.2174/138161211798764942

[119] Sanchez-Rodriguez MA, Zacarias-Flores M, Castrejon-Delgado L, Ruiz-Rodríguez AK, Mendoza-Nunez VM. Effects of hormone therapy on oxidative stress in postmenopausal women with metabolic syndrome. International Journal of Molecular Sciences. 2016;**17**:1388. DOI: 10.3390/ijms17091388

[120] Massafra C, Gioia D, De Felice C, Picciolini E, De Leo V, Bonifazi M, Bernabei A. Effects of estrogens and androgens on erythrocyte antioxidant superoxide dismutase, catalase and glutathione peroxidase activities during the menstrual cycle. Journal of Endocrinology. 2000;**167**(3):447-452. DOI: 0022-0795/00/0167-447

[121] Mumford SL, Browne RW, Schliep KC, Schmelzer J, Plowden TC, Michels KA, Sjaarda LA, Zarek SM, Perkins NJ, Messer LC, Radin RG, Wactawski-Wende J, Schisterman E. Serum antioxidants are associated with serum reproductive hormones and ovulation among healthy women. Journal of Nutrition. 2016;**146**:98-106. DOI: 10.3945/jn.115.217620

[122] Lutoslawska G, Tkaczyk J, Panczenko-Kresowska B, Hubner-Wozniak E, Skierska E, Gajewski AK. Plasma TBARS, blood GSH concentrations, and erythrocyte antioxidant enzyme activities in regularly menstruating women with ovulatory and anovulatory menstrual cycles. Clinica Chimica Acta. 2003;**331**(1-2):159-163. DOI: 10.1016/S0009-8981(03)00085-8

[123] Cornelli U, Belcaro G, Rosaria M, Cesarone MR, Finco A. Analysis of oxidative stress during the menstrual cycle. Reproductive Biology and Endocrinology. 2013;**11**(1):74. DOI: 10.1186/1477-7827-11-74

[124] Iida T, Inoue K, Ito Y, Ishikawa H, Kagiono M, Teradaira R, Chikamura C, Harada T, Ezoe S, Yatsuya H. Comparison of urinary levels of 8-hydroxy-2′-deoxyguanosine between young females with and without depressive symptoms during different menstrual phases. Acta Medica Okayama. 2015;**69**(1):45-50

[125] Chung SC, Goldfarb AH, Jamurtas AZ, Hegde SS, Lee J. Effect of exercise during the follicular and luteal phases on indices of oxidative stress in healthy women. Medicine and Science in Sports and Exercise. 1999;**31**(3):409-413. DOI: 10.1097/00005768-1999 03000-00009

[126] Bell HK, Bloomer RJ. Impact of serum estradiol on postprandial lipemia, oxidative stress, and inflammation across a single menstrual cycle. Gender Medicine. 2010;**7**(2):166-178. DOI: 10.1016/j.genm.2010.03.001

[127] Brunelli E, Domanico F, La Russa D, Pellegrino D. Sex differences in oxidative stress biomarkers. Current Drug Targets. 2014;**15**(8):811-815. DOI: 10.2174/1389450115666140624112317

[128] Kowalska K, Milnerowicz H. Pro/antioxidant status in young healthy women using oral contraceptives. Environmental Toxicology and Pharmacology. 2016;**43**:1-6. DOI: 10.1016/j.etap.2016.02.006

[129] Kanaley JA, Ji LL. Antioxidant enzyme activity during prolonged exercise in amenorrheic and eumenorrheic athletes. Metabolism. 1991;**40**(1):88-92. DOI: 10.1016/0026-0495(91)90197-5

[130] Akova B, Surmen-Gur E, Gur H, Dirican M, Sarandol E, Kucukoglu S. Exercise-induced oxidative stress and muscle performance in healthy women: Role of vitamin E supplementation and endogenous oestradiol. European Journal of Applied Physiology. 2001;**84**:141-147

[131] Klapcinska B, Sadowska-Krepa E, Manowska B, Pilis W, Sobczak A, Danch A. Effects of a low carbohydrate diet and graded exercise during the follicular and luteal phases on the blood antioxidant status in healthy women. European Journal of Applied Physiology. 2002;**87**(4-5):373-380. DOI: 10.1007/s00421-002-0641-1

[132] Samsudeen N, Rajagopalan A. Effect of different phases of menstrual cycle on cardio-respiratory efficiency in normal, overweight and obese female undergraduate students. Journal of Clinical and Diagnostic Research. 2016;**10**(12):CC01-CC04. DOI: 10.7860/JCDR/2016/23080.8954

[133] Abdollahpor A, Khosravi N, Zahra NR. Effects of the menstrual cycle phase on the blood lactate responses and exercise performance in active women. European Journal of Experimental Biology. 2013;**3**(3):206-210

[134] Pestana ER, Salvador EP, Pereira GB, Mostarda CT, Leite RD, Silva CR, Carvalho WRG. Influence of the mid-follicular and late luteal phases on anaerobic power in university students. Sport Sciences for Health. 2017;**13**:281-286. DOI: 10.1007/s11332-016-0344-3

[135] Bruinvels G, Burden RJ, McGregor AJ, Ackerman KE, Dooley M, Richards T, Pedlar C. Sport, exercise and the menstrual cycle: Where is the research? British Journal of Sports Medicine. 2017;**51**(6):487-488. DOI: 10.1136/bjsports-2016-096279

# Chapter 6

# Premature Ovarian Insufficiency

Abdelhamid Benmachiche and
Amel Dammene Debbih

Additional information is available at the end of the chapter

http://dx.doi.org/10.5772/intechopen.80090

**Abstract**

Premature ovarian insufficiency (POI) is a heterogeneous disorder, affecting approximately 1% of women before the age of 40. Heterogeneity of POI is reflected by various causes. The known causes are genetic defects, autoimmune ovarian damage, metabolic, iatrogenic following surgery, cancer therapy, and environmental factors. However, in most cases, the cause remains unknown (idiopathic POI). The main symptom is the absence of regular menstrual cycles, and the diagnosis is confirmed by the raised gonadotropins and low estradiol. The disorder usually leads to infertility and has long-term comorbidities such as cardiovascular diseases, osteoporosis, and cognitive impairments. Management includes the use of hormone replacement therapy till the age of natural menopause. In women having fertility issues, the spontaneous conception varies between 5 and 10%, and in vitro fertilization with donor oocytes remains the treatment of choice. Moreover, fertility preservation options can be offered to some patients with cancer and those at risk of early menopause, such as those with familial cases of POI. Further research is clearly needed, to identify new mechanisms which may improve the prediction of the early onset of the disease.

**Keywords:** premature ovarian insufficiency, irregular menstrual cycle, estrogen deficiency, hormone replacement therapy, infertility treatment

## 1. Introduction

Premature ovarian insufficiency (POI) is a heterogeneous condition defined by the presence of menopausal-level serum gonadotropins in repeated blood tests with menstrual disturbance (oligomenorrhea or amenorrhea) in adolescent girls or women under 40 years of age [1]. Several different terms have been used to describe this condition, such as premature menopause, premature ovarian insufficiency (POI), or premature ovarian failure (POF). Confusion exists concerning nomenclature, namely, the use of POF or POI. The term POI has been adopted recently by the European Society of Human Reproduction and Embryology (ESHRE) consensus instead of "failure" [2]. Because it was found to more accurately describe the fluctuating nature of the condition. The POF is best considered as the only final stage of POI [3, 4]. The incidence of spontaneous POI has been estimated to affect 1 in 100 women before 40 years of age and 1 in 1000 women before 30 years of age [1, 5]. Although the incidence of spontaneous POI appears to have remained stable, of increasing concern is the rising incidence of iatrogenic POI [6]. Improved survival following malignant diseases has led to increasing numbers of women experiencing the long-term effects of cancer treatments. A recent cohort study estimated the incidence of POI, both spontaneous and iatrogenic, at 7.4% [7]. The risk of POI varies by ethnicity, ranging from 0.1% in Japanese to 1% in Caucasian and 1.4% in African American and Hispanic groups [8]. Environmental factors such as cigarette smoking and poverty were associated with an increased risk of idiopathic POI. In contrast, certain factors related to ovulation, such as late menarche, irregular menstruation, and longer breastfeeding seem to reduce the risk of POI [9]. The familial form of POI is rare, representing 4–31% of all cases of POI [10–12]. Morris DH et al. (2011) reported that women were around six times more likely to have early menopause if their mother (odd ratio [OR], 6.2; $p < 0.001$) or older sister (OR, 5.5; $p < 0.001$) also experienced early menopause [13].

## 2. Objective

In this comprehensive review, we aim to provide an overview of the current knowledge of the identifiable causes leading to POI development and the recent advances in the management of its consequences in terms of long-term complications as well as in terms of infertility concerns.

## 3. Methods

*Literature search strategy*: Using the MEDLINE database and Google Scholar, we conducted a comprehensive literature search to identify relevant publications on menstrual cycle disorders associated with premature ovarian insufficiency. The keyword combinations include "premature ovarian insufficiency," "primary ovarian failure," "hypergonadotropic amenorrhea," "hypergonadotropic hypogonadism," and "early menopause."

*Selection criteria*: The search was restricted to articles that were published up to May 2018 in English language and that assessed at least one of the following aspects of the condition: "epidemiology," "diagnosis," "etiology," "long-term consequences," "hormonal replacement therapy," "infertility management," and "prediction."

*Data synthesis and analysis*: The conclusions and the interpretation of the findings were based on our personal experience. In addition, we provided some clinical recommendations and guidelines about the management of patients experiencing premature or early menopause based on the expertise of prestigious scientific societies such as the European Society for Human Reproduction and Embryology (ESHRE) and the American Society for Reproductive Medicine (ASRM). Statistical testing was not conducted.

## 4. Diagnosis

Current studies have failed to determine specific biomarkers or signs/symptoms of POI that will accurately predict when menopause will occur. Some women with POI may not experience any specific symptoms particularly in the idiopathic form of the largest etiology, which may delay the establishment of the diagnosis.

One study reported that over 50% of patients with POI had seen at least three clinicians before the diagnosis was made, and in 25% the diagnosis took more than 5 years [14]. Before puberty, the clinical picture is characterized by absent menarche, and pubertal delay results in absent sexual maturation. After puberty, the typical disorder is characterized by the loss of menstrual regularity (oligomenorrhea or amenorrhea) in young women for 3 or more consecutive months and often associated with symptoms of estrogen deficiency such as vasomotor symptoms which are similar to those observed with the onset of menopause, such as hot flushes, insomnia, nervousness, irritability, loss of libido, vaginal dryness, dyspareunia, etc. Female infertility is a common concern, as only 5–10% of the patients will conceive spontaneously [15]. POI may be part of other syndromic features: autoimmune polyendocrinopathy-candidiasis-ectodermal dystrophy, blepharophimosis-ptosis-epicanthus inversus syndrome, carbohydrate-deficient glycoprotein syndromes, galactosemia, Turner syndrome, and PHP I [16].

Additionally, patients can experience long-term consequences of hypoestrogenism, including low bone density (osteoporosis) [17], cardiovascular diseases [18], and neurocognitive disorders [19]. For the biochemical confirmation, follicle-stimulating hormone (FSH) levels are used as the gold standard in establishing a diagnosis of POI. Two serum FSH levels in the menopausal range should be obtained at least a month apart (**BOX 1**) [27]. However, there is a lack of consensus on adequate cutoff levels used to define hypergonadotropism. No follicles were found in ovarian biopsies when FSH levels are above 33 and 40 mIU/ml in women with primary and secondary amenorrhea, respectively [20]. Some women with POI express FSH levels lower than these proposed cutoff values, particularly women with autoantibodies. La Marca et al. (2009) found that women with POI due to steroidogenic cell autoimmunity had significantly lower FSH levels (n = 26, median 37 mIU/ml) compared with idiopathic POI (median 99 mIU/ml) (P = 0.001) [21]. Furthermore, estradiol (E2) levels are typically low, with a level of 50 pg/ml in women with absent or nonfunctioning follicles [22]. Antimullerian hormone (AMH) is currently the most convenient predictor of ovarian reserve. Very low AMH levels seem to play a role in predicting age at menopause [23, 24].

Younger than 40 years of age

Oligo/amenorrhea for at least 4 months

Two FSH levels in the menopausal range, obtained at least a month apart

Data from [27].

**Box 1.** Criteria to establish the diagnosis of premature ovarian insufficiency.

| Test | Implications | |
|---|---|---|
| | Positive test | Negative test |
| **Genetic/Chromosomal** | | |
| Karyotyping<br>(for diagnosis of Turner syndrome) | Refer to endocrinologist, cardiologist and geneticist | A second analysis of the karyotype in epithelial cells (in case of high clinical suspicion) |
| Test for Y-chromosomal material | Discuss gonadectomy with the patient | |
| Fra-X | Refer to geneticist | |
| Autosomal genetic testing[1] | | |
| **Antibodies2** | | |
| ACA/21OH antibodies | Refer to endocrinologist | Re-test in case of clinical signs |
| TPO-Ab | Test TSH every year | or symptoms |

[1]not at present indicated in women with POI, unless there is evidence suggesting a specific mutation (e.g. BPES).
[2]POI of unknown cause or if an immune disorder is suspected.
Data from [25].

**Table 1.** Summary of diagnostic workup.

The differential diagnosis is based on the exclusion of other causes of primary and secondary amenorrhea, for example, pregnancy, polycystic ovarian syndrome, hypothalamic-pituitary disease (pituitary tumors, hyperprolactinemia, Kallmann syndrome), hypothalamic amenorrhea (induced by stress, intensive exercise, anorexia, weight loss, fasting, and severe diseases), endocrine disorders (hyperthyroidism, hypothyroidism, and Cushing syndrome), and vaginal/uterus anatomical abnormalities, such as Rokitansky syndrome or Asherman syndrome. Once the diagnosis has been confirmed, second-line investigations to look for an underlying cause should be considered which may have implications for the individualization of the management **Table 1** [25].

## 5. Etiology

Three potential mechanisms can be associated with POI, that is, a congenital decrease in primordial follicles, accelerated follicular atresia, and an inability to recruit primordial follicles [26]. The known causes of POI are wide ranging and can be divided into spontaneous and iatrogenic categories.

### 5.1. Spontaneous POI

Most cases of spontaneous POI are idiopathic despite the diagnostic advances [27] but may be also due to genetic causes, autoimmune disorders, metabolic dysfunction, enzyme deficiencies, toxins, or infections [27–29].

#### *5.1.1. Genetic causes of POI*

The normal ovarian function requires the presence of many intact genes functionally normally and in a coordinated fashion. Chromosomal abnormalities are found in around 10–12% of women with POI, of which the majority is X chromosomal abnormalities [30]. An increasing number of studies have documented autosomal involvement. The incidence of chromosomal abnormalities is higher in women with primary amenorrhea (21%) than in those presenting with secondary amenorrhea (11%) [31].

##### *5.1.1.1. X Chromosome defects*

Both the short and long arms of the X chromosome appear to play important roles.

X Chromosome defects usually involve either complete deletion of one X (Turner syndrome) or partial deletions, duplications, and balanced translocations between the X and autosomal chromosomes. Females lacking an X chromosome as well as those showing an extra X chromosome are predisposed to developing POI. Monosomy X (45X), known as Turner syndrome, is due to the loss of the second sex chromosome and affects 1 in 2500 live-born female infants and has a frequency of 4–5% in POI [32]. In phenotypic women, Turner syndrome is associated with short stature, gonadal dysgenesis, and primary amenorrhea. In women with Tuner syndrome, oocyte loss usually begins early in childhood as a result of accelerated follicle atresia [33]. The vast majority of pregnancies with this karyotype end in spontaneous miscarriage, and it is argued that the surviving individuals most likely carry some degree of mosaicism [34]. In mosaic Turner syndrome (45X/46XX), patients have a milder phenotype and may present later with secondary amenorrhea and hypergonadotropic hypogonadism. Trisomy X (47XXX) is caused by nondisjunction of the X chromosome during meiosis. It is the most common form of aneuploidy, occurring in 1:900 women. About 1.5–3.8% patients with POI had the triple X [30, 35] and may manifest in many mosaic forms, that is, 45X/47XXX, 46XX/47XXX, or 47XXX/48XXXX [36]. The presence of three X chromosomes presumably leads to meiotic disturbance and, secondarily, ovarian failure. X Chromosome deletions associated with POI are more common than translocations. At present, the microdeletions are not normally identified by conventional karyotyping and so often go unrecognized. Krauss et al. reported in 1987 a family in which one woman and two girls, with early menopause, had a deletion of the long arm of the X chromosome (Xq21–Xq27) [37]. Cytogenetic and molecular analyses of POI women carrying a balanced X-autosome translocation allowed the identification of a "critical region" for the ovarian development and function on the long arm of the X chromosome from Xq13.3 to q27. Various deletions or translocations occurring within this region and also on the short arm of the X chromosome have been associated with POI [38, 39]. POI can also be associated with the Xq isochromosome which occurs when the centromere splits abnormally in the transverse plane instead of the longitudinal plane. The resulting chromosome pair contains structurally identical arms with identical genes. The isochromosome for the long arm (q) is the most common X structural abnormality. These patients present with streak gonads and Turner-like characteristics which are rare causes of POI [40].

### *5.1.1.2. Single-gene defects*

The fragile X syndrome is an X-linked dominant genetic disorder that is a leading cause of mental retardation and autism. Women exhibiting extended repeats of the CGG trinucleotide sequence may be classified as having the permutation (55–199 repeats) or the full condition (>200 repeats). There is an association, although nonlinear, between the number of repeats and the severity of the condition. The fragile site of the X chromosome contains a (CGG) repeat in the 5′ region of the gene. In normal variants, the trinucleotide repeat ranges from 6 to 55 repeats.

The syndrome occurs when the number of the repeats exceeds 200, being denominated as full mutation alleles. The fragile X mental retardation 1 (FMR1) gene premutation, mapped at position Xq27.3 on the X chromosome, is the most frequently identified single-gene mutation associated with POI outside the Xq POI critical region. It has been shown that females carrying a premutation have up to 23% rate of POI and experience menopause 5 years earlier than average [41]. The FMR1 premutation has been identified in 11% of familial POI and 3% of sporadic cases [42–44], and therefore, screening for the FMR1 premutation is usually recommended in women diagnosed with POI to identify those patients and family members who may be at risk of having children with fragile X syndrome. Those with identified premutation should be referred for family genetic counseling. *The bone morphogenetic protein 15 gene (*BMP15*) is a member of transforming growth factor beta (TGF-ß) superfamily and is located on the short arm of the X chromosome (Xp11.2) within the Xp POI critical region* [45, 46]. It is an *oocyte-specific folliculogenesis growth differentiation factor (GDF) and appears to have a vital role in folliculogenesis and granulosa cell growth.*

Approximately 1.5–12% of POI is associated with *BMP15* gene mutation [47–50].

Fragile site, folic acid type, rare (*FRAXE*)/fragile site mental retardation 2 gene (*FMR2*) has been described in patients who have the cytogenetic changes of fragile X syndrome but who are *FMR1* mutation negative. It was found at Xq28 and found to be folate sensitive [51].

### *5.1.1.3. Autosomal genetic defects*

While several genes relevant to ovarian function lie on the X chromosome, autosomal genes also appear to be involved in the development of POI [26].

In recent years, attention has focused on genes that are known to play a role in folliculogenesis and ovarian function. Oocyte-specific gene expression is necessary for primordial follicle formation and their subsequent differentiation into primary follicles. A number of autosomal genes have been suggested as a causative factor of POI. For some of these genes, mutations are identified, while others are listed as candidate genes with a need for further investigation. The genes with identified mutations that could result in POI are genes involved in folliculogenesis (NR5A1, NOBOX, FIGLA, and FOXL2), folliculogenesis growth factors (GDF9 and inhibin A), sex hormone function (*CYP17A1*, *CYP19*, FSH/luteinizing hormone (LH) receptors, and *NR5A1*) [26, 38], or genes identified in syndromes often associated with POI such as Bloom syndrome BLM 15q26.1 [52], Ataxia telangiectasia,

A-T. ATM 11q22-q23 [53], Werner syndrome WRN 8p12 [54], and Rothmund-Thomson syndrome RTS 8q24.3 [55]. Given that the conventional approaches have had limited success in finding causative genes, further research and new techniques on the genetic background of POI including genome-wide analysis in affected families may change this recommendation in the near future.

### *5.1.2. Autoimmune causes of POI*

Anti-ovarian antibodies are reported in POI by several studies, but their specificity and pathogenic role are questionable. Autoimmune diseases are estimated to be involved in the pathogenesis of up to 5% of POI cases. Adrenal autoimmunity is thought to account for 60–80% of autoimmune POI [56], and there is a strong association between the presence of adrenal antibodies and a diagnosis of autoimmune lymphocytic oophoritis [57]. The evidence of oophoritis is rare (<3%) in POI in the absence of adrenal involvement [16]. The presence of many other autoantibodies has been investigated such as ovarian and other steroidogenic cell autoantibodies; however, reliable markers to diagnose non-adrenal autoimmunity are yet to be identified [56]. POI can be associated with endocrine (thyroid, hypoparathyroid, diabetes mellitus, and hypophysitis) and non-endocrine diseases (chronic candidiasis, idiopathic thrombocytopenic purpura, vitiligo, alopecia, autoimmune hemolytic anemia, pernicious anemia, systemic lupus erythematosus (SLE), rheumatoid arthritis, Crohn's disease, Sjogren syndrome, primary biliary cirrhosis, and chronic active hepatitis) (**Table 2**) [16, 58, 59]. POI may be part of the autoimmune polyglandular syndromes (APS) when accompanied by other autoimmune endocrinopathies. POI is more common with APS types I and III than with APS type II [60].

### *5.1.3. Metabolic causes of POI*

A number of inherited enzymatic pathway disorders have been associated with ovarian follicular dysfunction leading to POI such as galactose-1-phosphate uridylyltransferase deficiency (galactosemia) [61], 19, carbohydrate-deficient glycoprotein deficiency [62], 17α-hydroxylase/17,20 desmolase deficiency [63], and aromatase mutations [64] where there is biochemical damage of the ovary and autoimmune regulator which triggers autoimmune damage. However, the strength of evidence linking each anomaly with POI is variable.

| | |
|---|---|
| Endocrine | Hypo/hyperthyroidism, Hypoparathyroidism, Diabetes mellitus type II, Hypophysitis, Addison's disease. |
| Non-endocrine | Idiopathic thrombocytemic purpura, Chronic candidiasis, Vitiligo, Alopecia, Hemolytic or Pernicious anemia, |
| | Systemic lupus erythematodes, Rheumatoid arthritis, Cirrhosis, Sjogren's sy, Primary biliary cirrhosis, Chronic hepatitis etc. |

Data from [16, 58, 59].

**Table 2.** Endocrine and non-endocrine diseases associated with premature ovarian failure.

### 5.2. Induced POI

The induced POI may result from damage to the ovaries, such as that caused by iatrogenic agents like chemotherapy, radiotherapy, pelvic surgery, and also environmental toxic agents.

#### *5.2.1. Cancer therapy*

There is an overall increase in cancer prevalence followed by an increase in long-term survival of the affected patients these days compared to the past. The 5-year survival rate for childhood, adolescent, and young adult cancer currently exceeds 80% [65]. Medical treatment for neoplastic conditions can be associated with POI. Chemotherapy and radiotherapy are well-documented causes of POI.

Chemotherapy induces apoptosis of mature ovarian follicles, and histological studies have shown fibrosis, vascular damage, and reduced follicle numbers. The gonadotoxic effect of chemotherapy is drug and dose dependent [66]. Alkylating agents have been shown to be gonadotoxic [67]. The prepubertal ovary is relatively resistant to this form of gonadotoxicity [67]. The risk of developing POI after radiotherapy is dependent on the radiation therapy field (abdominal pelvic, total body irradiation) and on dose and age [68–70]. Transposition of the ovaries in young women requiring pelvic irradiation helps in preserving their ovarian function.

#### *5.2.2. Pelvic surgery*

Aside from surgical menopause due to bilateral oophorectomy, limited evidence suggests that pelvic surgery is maybe associated with POI such as hysterectomy [71], tubal sterilization [72], or both ovarian surgery for endometrioma and endometriosis [73] presumably due to damage to ovarian blood vessels as a result of the surgical procedure. Research has now also linked ovarian drilling for polycystic ovary syndrome and removal of endometriotic cysts to an earlier age at menopause [74, 75].

#### *5.2.3. Toxins*

The increasing prevalence of POI in recent years might be also due to an increase in presently unidentified environmental toxic agents. However, studies examining the cause and effect of the chemical substances and POI in humans are rare.

Chang et al. (2007) found that cigarette smoking was associated with an increased risk of POI (OR = 1.82 [1.03–3.23]) [76]. Many other endocrine-disrupting substances have been also suggested to be ovotoxic and influencing the age of menopause such as 2-bromopropane [76], vinylcyclohexene diepoxide (VCD) [77], polycyclic aromatic hydrocarbons (PAHs) [77], etc., but they are not readily considered as diagnosable causes of POI. Further research is warranted to clarify in which toxicants affect human reproduction and how insufficiency with FSH values is found in the menopausal range [78].

#### *5.2.4. Infections*

It has been indicated that many viral infections can be followed by POI, but only mumps oophoritis has been directly linked to POI, explaining 3–7% of POI cases [79]. Other potential causes of POI include tuberculosis, malaria, varicella, and *Shigella* [80]. More recently, there has been suggestion that human immunodeficiency virus (HIV) infection (or antiviral therapy) can lead to POI. However, a recent systematic review revealed nonconclusive evidence due to a significant methodological limitation with available data [81].

## 6. Management

Patients must be provided with adequate information (education, understanding, and counseling). Management should address the following aspects: psychology support, ovarian hormone replacement for the prevention of long-term complications, and therapy for fertility.

### 6.1. Psychologic support

The diagnosis of POI is an extremely devastating psychologic disturbance [35]. Some will experience a range of emotions such as high levels of depression and low levels of self-esteem with negative effects on sexuality [82], and providers should offer support regarding infertility, altered self-image, and sexual dysfunction. Patients may benefit from referral to a psychologist and support groups [83].

### 6.2. Hormone replacement therapy

Hormone replacement therapy (HRT) remains the cornerstone of treatment for relief of menopausal symptoms (including vasomotor instability, sexual dysfunction, mood, fatigue, and skin issues) and prevention of long-term morbidity and earlier mortality related to prolonged estrogen deficiency [84]. The results of Women's Health Initiative (WHI) study should not be applied to young women with POI [85, 86]. In contrast with women older than 50s, POI is a pathologic condition in which young women have low serum E2 levels compared with their peers. For young women with E2 deficiency, hormone therapy is indeed a "replacement," whereas in women with normal menopause, hormone therapy is hormone "extension." Physiological replacement of ovarian steroid hormones until the age of 50 years (the average age of natural menopause) is generally accepted as routine, unless a specific contraindication exists, such as an estrogen-dependent malignancy. At present, very little evidence exists regarding the optimum method of hormone replacement, and options include both the combined oral contraceptive pill (COC) and hormone replacement. Data regarding the optimal estradiol levels in POI are lacking; however, the average serum estradiol level during the menstrual cycle in normal women is approximately 100 pg/ml [87]. Transdermal and transvaginal replacement of 100 μg/day of estradiol achieves physiologic blood levels in this range and provides adequate symptomatic relief. The transdermal route has the advantage of avoidance of first-pass hepatic metabolism and appears to be free of an excess risk of thrombosis compared with oral estrogen [88–90]. To reduce the risk of endometrial hyperplasia, 5–10 mg of medroxyprogesterone acetate should be given for 12 days of the month, provided that the uterus is present and intact [90, 91]. However, the optimum type of progestogen is unclear. With the use of this regimen, most of women will develop monthly withdrawal bleeding, which may be psychologically important to the patient. The COC is also commonly used as hormone replacement in POI. However, they should not be recommended as first-line hormone replacement. Indeed, they result in supraphysiological doses of sex steroid hormones and are associated with an increased risk of thromboembolic events related to the first-pass effect on the liver [27]. Androgen replacement could be carefully considered for women who have persistent fatigue and low libido despite optimized estrogen replacement [92]. Transdermal testosterone administration and dehydroepiandrosterone treatment are two of the options for androgen replacement in these women [93]. Importantly, this should be performed with great caution and for relatively short periods until more data are available. When there has been no spontaneous start to puberty or progression of breast development, many options for HRT are suggested for puberty induction. However, systemic administration of increasing doses of estradiol, preferably by transdermal application, is the only form of therapy to achieve natural levels of estradiol in blood and mimic normal estradiol physiology in adolescence and adulthood [94, 95]. Patients who do not want to get pregnant should be offered contraception due to the 5–10% chance of spontaneous conception. Women with untreated POI are at increased risk of developing long-term comorbidities such as cardiovascular disease [96], metabolic syndrome [97], osteoporosis, dementia, cognitive impairment, Parkinsonism, reduced sexual function, and psychological well-being. Untreated POI can induce specific increase in mortality rate due to complications of the prolonged estrogen deficiency compared to those with a menopause after the age of 50 years [98]. The main reason for shortened life expectancy in women with POI is cardiovascular disease. The Framingham study was one of the first to show a higher incidence of cardiovascular disease among postmenopausal women than age-matched women who were premenopausal [99]. A number of studies have subsequently demonstrated higher rates of coronary artery disease, higher rates of heart failure, and higher rates of mortality in women reaching menopause before 40–45 years of age, and it has been demonstrated that this impairment was reversed by estrogen replacement [100]. Compared with control women, women with premature ovarian insufficiency have reduced bone mineral density. The prevalence of osteoporosis in POI appears to be in the range of 8–14% [101]. Multiple studies have shown that the lower bone mineral density (BMD) seen in women with POI is associated with significantly higher overall fracture risk, and this has been associated with the presence, degree, and duration of estrogen deficiency. Studies on fracture risk in early menopause compared to natural menopause have demonstrated that fracture rates are reduced among women with POI or early menopause who are treated with the use of HRT [101–103]. Early data demonstrate an increased risk of cognitive impairment [104]. Some studies suggest that estrogen is neuroprotective. The Mayo Clinic Cohort Study of Oophorectomy and Aging demonstrated that women who underwent either unilateral or bilateral oophorectomy before the onset of the menopause had an increased risk of cognitive impairment or dementia [105] and Parkinsonism [104] compared to controls and that this risk increased with younger age at oophorectomy. They also demonstrated a protective role for estrogen replacement in women with bilateral oophorectomy when taken until at least 50 years of age. A similar finding was noted in a Danish cohort study, revealing an increased risk of dementia in women undergoing oophorectomy prior to the age of 50 years, with a similar trend of increasing risk with earlier age at oophorectomy [106].

http://dx.doi.org/10.5772/intechopen.80090

### 6.3. Fertility

#### *6.3.1. Spontaneous conception and POI*

For many women with POI, infertility is the most devastating aspect of the diagnosis.

Fertility of women with POI is severely diminished, but unlike menopause, POI may be accompanied with spontaneous ovarian activity and natural pregnancies in approximately 5–10% [107]. Currently, no fertility treatment has been found to effectively increase fertility in women with POI including estrogens [108–110], 5-dehydroepiandrosterone (DHEA) [111], corticosteroids [112], and azathioprine [113].

#### *6.3.2. Assisted reproductive technology (ART) and POI*

##### *6.3.2.1. Oocyte donation*

The only proven therapy for obtaining a pregnancy in patients with POI is fertilization of a donor oocyte. At present IVF with donor oocytes confers the highest chance of pregnancy for women with POI with high success rates of around 40–50% per cycle.

The pregnancy rate from oocyte donation is not greatly affected by the recipient's age [114, 115].

##### *6.3.2.2. Fertility management of the Turner syndrome*

There are special considerations regarding oocyte donation in women with Turner syndrome. If pregnancy is desired, hormone replacement therapy can be initiated to increase uterine size, followed by assisted reproductive technology, namely, in vitro fertilization with an oocyte donor. However, coexisting cardiac abnormalities associated with Turner syndrome may increase the risk of pregnancy for the mother, and therefore this type of approach to achieve pregnancy is strongly discouraged [116, 117]. Should a Y chromosome be identified with or without an SRY gene mutation, the patient should be counseled about the risk of development of a gonadal tumor, and gonadectomy should be advised [118, 119].

##### *6.3.2.3. Fertility preservation and POI*

Fertility preservation may also be considered for women at risk of POI; in young women who require cancer treatments, including chemotherapy, radiotherapy, and surgery; or for those who have a strong family history of POI. Options for fertility preservation include ovarian transposition, oocyte or embryo cryopreservation, and ovarian tissue cryopreservation. Ovarian transposition remains the standard of care for women undergoing pelvic radiation, although it has been suggested that it may be combined with ovarian tissue cryopreservation. Embryo cryopreservation remains the most successful technique, with success rates approaching that of fresh embryo transfer [120, 121]. Live birth rates of approximately 30% per embryo transfer have been reported, depending on the age of the patient [120]. The success of oocyte cryopreservation has also improved significantly in recent years, and birth rates similar to that of fresh oocytes have been reported [122]. Oocyte cryopreservation is a potential option for women without a partner. Since the initial report of successful pregnancy following ovarian tissue cryopreservation and subsequent transplant in 2000 [123], there has been increasing success with the technique [124, 125].

## 7. Prediction and genetic counseling

Contrary to the induced POI occurring in cancer survivors, the spontaneous POI particularly the idiopathic form is still difficult to be predicted in the general population. Low circulating AMH level is currently thought to be the most reliable measure of reduced ovarian reserve and may play a role in predicting age at menopause [23]. Sowers et al. (2008) have shown that AMH starts declining 5 years before the final menstrual period. All these observations suggest a potential role for AMH in screening women at high risk for POI and in well woman screening programs [24]. Autoantibody screening, for anti-adrenal, anti-ovarian, and antithyroid antibodies, is also recommended [25]. Genetic counseling is nowadays recommended for several reasons, when a genetic form of POI is suspected or identified. The prevalence of familial POI has been reported to be between 4 and 31% of cases in various series [126–129]. The early diagnosis of familial POI will provide the opportunity to predict the likelihood of early menopause and allow other reproductive choices to be made, such as freezing embryos or having children earlier. Karyotyping and screening for the FMR1 gene permutation are especially important in younger patients with or without mental retardation or when a female is born from a family with female members affected with POI. The review of McConkie-Rosell states that approximately 13–24% of women who are fragile X premutation carriers (identified through families with fragile X syndrome) have POI [130].

## 8. Future

Continued advances in DNA sequencing techniques will facilitate finding additional genes responsible for POI in other portions of the genome. Besides, the future holds the possibility of restoring ovarian function with ovarian or oogonial stem cell (OSC) therapy which may open the door to novel fertility preservation strategies for women with both age-related and POI [131]. More recently, Kawamura et al. (2013) have successfully promoted follicle growth, retrieved mature oocytes, and performed IVF. Following embryo transfer, a healthy baby was delivered [132]. This in vitro activation (IVA) approach has been reproduced by a group in Zhengzhou University, China, with two cases [133]. Up to the summer of 2018, there were more than one dozen of successful cases.

## 9. Summary

The POI represents a continuum of declining ovarian function with intermittent ovulation in women below the age of 40 years resulting usually in an earlier than average menopause. Its incidence is gradually increasing secondary to the improved survival of young women with cancer. In most cases, the etiology is unknown, but known causes include genetic disorders, particularly involving the X chromosome, associations with autoimmune diseases, cancer therapy, pelvic surgery, and also environmental toxic agents. A timely diagnosis of POI is the main challenge. The typical disorder is characterized by the loss of regular menstrual cycles, and the diagnosis is confirmed by the detection of menopausal-level serum gonadotropins in repeated blood tests. Second-line investigations should be directed by specific clinical indications. Regardless of the etiology, patients with POI are estrogen deficient. The aims of HRT extend beyond simply symptom relief to levels that support cardiovascular, bone, and cognitive health. Only 5–10% of women with POI may conceive spontaneously. Currently, there are no proven treatments to improve ovarian function, and only the use of donor eggs with IVF confers the highest chance of pregnancy. However, in women with Turner syndrome, this approach is strongly discouraged. To date, the prediction of POI is difficult in the general population. However, in women at risk of POI particularly those who have a strong family history of POI, or require cancer treatments, a screening program will provide the opportunity to predict the likelihood of early onset menopause and to consider fertility preservation as well. Further research is needed particularly in idiopathic POI to identify mechanisms and specific molecular defects which may offer a better opportunity for early therapeutic interventions.

## Conflicts of interest

There are no conflicts of interest.

## Financial support and sponsorship

Nil.

## Author details

Abdelhamid Benmachiche[1*] and Amel Dammene Debbih[2]

*Address all correspondence to: benmachiche@gmail.com

1 Center for Reproductive Medicine, Clinique Ibn Rochd, Constantine, Algeria,

2 Faculty of Medicine of Algiers, Bologhine University Hospital Center, Algiers, Algeria

## References

[1] Coulam CB, Adamson SC, Annegers JF. Incidence of premature ovarian failure. Obstetrics and Gynecology. 1986;**67**(4):604-606

[2] Webber L, Davies M, Anderson R, et al. ESHRE Guideline: Management of Women With Premature Ovarian Insufficiency. Grimbergen, Belgium: European Society of Human Reproduction and Embryology; 2015

[3] Welt CK. Primary ovarian insufficiency: A more accurate term for premature ovarian failure. Clinical Endocrinology. 2008;**68**:499-509

[4] Kalu E, Panay N. Spontaneous premature ovarian failure: Management challenges. Gynecological Endocrinology. 2008;**24**:273-279

[5] Sowers MF et al. Premature menopause in a multi-ethnic population study of the menopause transition. Human Reproduction. 2003;**18**:199-206

[6] Panay N, Fenton A. Premature ovarian failure: A growing concern. Climacteric. 2008; **11**:1-3

[7] Islam R, Cartwright R. The impact of premature ovarian failure on quality of life: Results from the UK 1958 Birth Cohort. Presented at: 27th Annual Meeting of ESHRE; 3-6 July 2011; Stockholm. Sweden

[8] Luborsky JL, Meyer P, Sowers MF, et al. Premature menopause in a multi-ethnic population study of the menopause transition. Human Reproduction. 2003;**18**:199-206

[9] Chang SH, Kim CS, Lee KS, et al. Premenopausal factors influencing premature ovarian failure and early menopause. Maturitas. 2007;**58**:19-30

[10] Conway GS, Kaltsas G, Patel A, Davies MC, Jacobs HS. Characterization of idiopathic premature ovarian failure. Fertility and Sterility. 1996;**64**:337-341

[11] Cramer DW, Xu H, Harlow BL. Family history as a predictor of early menopause. Fertility and Sterility. 1995;**64**:740-745

[12] Torgerson DJ, Thomas RE, Reid DM. Mothers and daughters menopausal ages: Is there a link? European Journal of Obstetrics, Gynecology, and Reproductive Biology. 1997;**74**:63-66

[13] Morris DH, Jones ME, Schoemaker MJ, Ashworth A, Swerdlow AJ. Familial concordance for age at natural menopause: Results from the breakthrough generations study. Menopause. 2011;**18**:956-961

[14] Alzubaidi NH, Chapin HL, Vanderhoof VH, et al. Meeting the needs of young women with secondary amenorrhea and spontaneous premature ovarian failure. Obstetrics and Gynecology. 2002;**99**:720-725

[15] McKinlay SM, Brambilla DJ, Posner JG. The normal menopause transition. Maturitas. 1992;**14**:103-115

[16] Hoek A, Schoemaker J, Drexhage HA. Premature ovarian failure and ovarian autoimmunity. Endocrine Reviews. 1997;**18**:107-134

[17] Gallagher JC. Effect of early menopause on bone mineral density and fractures. Menopause. 2007;**14**:567-571

[18] Atsma F, Bartelink ML, Grobbee DE, van der Schouw YT. Postmenopausal status and early menopause as independent risk factors for cardiovascular disease: A meta-analysis. Menopause. 2006;**13**:265-279

[19] van der Stege JG, Groen H, van Zadelhoff SJ, Lambalk CB, Braat DD, van Kasteren YM, et al. Decreased androgen concentrations and diminished general and sexual well-being in women with premature ovarian failure. Menopause. 2008;**15**:23-31

[20] Goldenberg RL, Grodin JM, Rodbard D, Ross GT. Gonadotropins in women with amenorrhea. The use of plasma follicle-stimulating hormone to differentiate women with and without ovarian follicles. American Journal of Obstetrics and Gynecology. 1973 Aug 1;**116**(7):1003-1012

[21] La Marca A, Marzotti S, Brozzetti A, Stabile G, Artenisio AC, Bini V, et al. Primary ovarian insufficiency due to steroidogenic cell autoimmunity is associated with a preserved pool of functioning follicles. The Journal of Clinical Endocrinology and Metabolism. 2009 Oct;**94**(10):3816-3823. DOI: 10.1210/jc.2009-0817. Epub 2009 Jul 21

[22] Rebar RW. Premature ovarian failure. Obstetrics and Gynaecology. 2009;**113**:1355-1363. DOI: 10.1097/AOG.0b013e3181a66843

[23] Tehrani A, Shakeri N, Azizi F. Whether age at menopause is predictable using serum anti-Mullerian hormone concentration? Human Reproduction. 2010;**25**:i1-i3

[24] Sowers MR, Eyvazzadeh AD, McConnell D, et al. Antimullerian hormone and inhibin B in the definition of ovarian aging and the menopause transition. The Journal of Clinical Endocrinology and Metabolism. 2008;**93**:3478-3483

[25] Webber L, Davies M, Anderson R, Bartlett J, Braat D, Cartwright B, et al. Vermeulen N ESHRE guideline: Management of women with premature ovarian insufficiency. European Society for Human Reproduction and Embryology (ESHRE) Guideline Group on POI. Human Reproduction. 2016 May;**31**(5):926-937

[26] Persani L, Rossetti R, Cacciatore C. Genes involved in human premature ovarian failure. Journal of Molecular Endocrinology. 2010;**45**:257-279

[27] Nelson LM. Clinical practice. Primary ovarian insufficiency. The New England Journal of Medicine. 2009;**360**:606-614

[28] North American Menopause Society. Menopause Practice: A Clinician's Guide. 3rd ed. Cleveland, OH: North American Menopause Society; 2007

[29] Santoro N. Mechanisms of premature ovarian failure. Annales d'Endocrinologie. 2003; **64**:87-92

[30] Kalantari H, Madani T, Zari Moradi S, Mansouri Z, Almadani N, Gourabi H, Mohseni Meybodi A. Cytogenetic analysis of 179 Iranian women with premature ovarian failure. Gynecological Endocrinology. 2013;**29**:588-591

[31] Jiao X, Qin C, Li J, Qin Y, Gao X, Zhang B, et al. Cytogenetic analysis of 531 Chinese women with premature ovarian failure. Human Reproduction. 2012;**7**:2201-2207

[32] Luisi S, Orlandini C, Regini C, Pizzo A, Vellucci F, Petraglia F. Premature ovarian management. Journal of Endocrinological Investigation. 2015;**38**:597-603

[33] Bianco B, Nunes Lipay MV, Guedes AD, Verreschi IT. Clinical implications of the detection of Y-chromosome mosaicism in Turner's syndrome: Report of 3 cases. Fertility and Sterility. 2008 Oct;**90**(4):1197.e17-1197.e20

[34] Hook EB, Warburton D. Turner syndrome revisited: Review of new data supports the hypothesis that all viable 45, X cases are cryptic mosaics with a rescue cell line, implying an origin by mitotic loss. Human Genetics. 2014;**133**(4):417-424

[35] Goswami R, Goswami D, Kabra M, Gupta N, Dubey S, Dadhwal V. Prevalence of the triple X syndrome in phenotypically normal women with premature ovarian failure and its association with autoimmune thyroid disorders. Fertility and Sterility. 2003;**4**:1052-1054

[36] Villanueva AL, Rebar RW. Triple-X syndrome and premature ovarian failure. Obstetrics and Gynecology. 1983;**62**(3 Suppl):70s-73s

[37] Krauss CM, Turksoy RN, Atkins L, Laughlin C, Brown LG, Page DC. Familial premature ovarian failure due to an inter-stitial deletion of the long arm of the X chromosome. The New England Journal of Medicine. 1987;**317**:125-131

[38] Zhao H, Chen ZJ. Genetic association studies in female reproduction: From candidate-gene approaches to genome-wide mapping. Molecular Human Reproduction. 2013;**19**: 644-654

[39] Cox L, Liu JH. Primary ovarian insufficiency: An update. International Journal of Women's Health. 2014;**6**:235-243

[40] Simpson JL. Gonadal dysgenesis and abnormalities of the human sex chromosomes: Current status of phenotypic-karyotypic correlations. Birth Defects Original Article Series. 1975;**11**:23-59

[41] Willemsen R, Levenga J, Oostra B. CGG repeat in the FMR1 gene: Size matters. Clinical Genetics. 2011;**80**:214-225

[42] Marozzi A, Vegetti W, Manfredini E, et al. Association between premature ovarian failure and fragile x premutation. Human Reproduction. 2000;**15**:197-202

[43] Murray A. Premature ovarian failure and the FMR1 gene. Seminars in Reproductive Medicine. 2000;**18**:59-66

[44] Bussani C, Papi L, Sestini R, et al. Premature ovarian failure and fragile X premutation: A study on 45 women. European Journal of Obstetrics, Gynecology, and Reproductive Biology. 2004;**112**:189-191

[45] Dube JL, Wang P, Elvin J, Lyons KM, Celeste AJ, Matzuk MM. The bone morphogenetic protein 15 gene is X-linked and expressed in oocytes. Molecular Endocrinology. 1998;**12**:1809-1817

[46] Aaltonen J, Laitinen MP, Vuojolainen K, Jaatinen R, Horelli-Kuitunen N, Seppa L, et al. Human growth differentiation factor 9 (GDF-9) and its novel homolog GDF-9B are

expressed in oocytes during early folliculogenesis. The Journal of Clinical Endocrinology and Metabolism. 1999;**84**:2744-2750

[47] Laissue P, Christin-Maitre S, Touraine P, et al. Mutations and sequence variants in GDF9 and BMP15 in patients with premature ovarian failure. European Journal of Endocrinology. 2006;**154**:739-744

[48] Di Pasquale E, Rossetti R, Marozzi A, et al. Identification of new variants of human BMP15 gene in a large cohort of women with premature ovarian failure. The Journal of Clinical Endocrinology and Metabolism. 2006;**91**:1976-1979

[49] Rossetti R, Di Pasquale E, Marozzi A, et al. BMP15 mutations associated with primary ovarian insufficiency cause a defective production of bioactive protein. Human Mutation. 2009;**30**:804-810

[50] Tiotiu D, Alvaro Mercadal B, Imbert R, et al. Variants of the BMP15 gene in a cohort of patients with premature ovarian failure. Human Reproduction. 2010;**25**:1581-1587

[51] Sutherland GR, Baker E. Characterisation of a new rare fragile site easily confused with the fragile X. Human Molecular Genetics. 1992;**1**:111-113

[52] Ellis NA, German J. Molecular genetics of Bloom's syndrome. Human Molecular Genetics. 1996;**5**:1457-1463

[53] Gatti RA, Boder E, Vinters HV, Sparkes RS, Norman A, Lange K. Ataxia-telangiectasia: An interdisciplinary approach to pathogenesis. Medicine. 1991;**2**:99-117

[54] Epstein CJ, Martin GM, Schultz AL, Motulsky AG. Werner's syndrome a review of its symptomatology, natural history, pathologic features, genetics and relationship to the natural aging process. Medicine. 1966;**3**:177-221

[55] Wang LL, Levy ML, Lewis RA, Chintagumpala MM, Lev D, Rogers M, et al. Clinical manifestations in a cohort of 41 Rothmund-Thomson syndrome patients. American Journal of Medical Genetics. 2001;**1**:11-17

[56] Silva CA, Yamakami LY, Aikawa NE, Araujo DB, Carvalho JF, Bonfa E. Autoimmune primary ovarian insufficiency. Autoimmunity Reviews. 2014;**13**:427-430

[57] Bakalov VK, Anasti JN, Calis KA, et al. Autoimmune oophoritis as a mechanism of follicular dysfunction in women with 46, XX spontaneous premature ovarian failure. Fertility and Sterility. 2005;**84**:958-965

[58] Rebar RW, Cedars MI. Hypergonadotrophic forms of amenorrhea in young women. Endocrinology and Metabolism Clinics of North America. 1992;**21**:173-191

[59] Betterle C, Dal Pra C, Mantero F, Zanchetta R. Autoimmune adrenal insufficiency and autoimmune polyendocrine syndromes: Autoantibodies, autoantigens, and their applicability in diagnosis and disease prediction. Endocrine Reviews. 2002;**23**:327-364

[60] Kauffman RP, Castracane VD. Premature ovarian failure associated with autoimmune polyglandular syndrome: Pathophysiological mechanisms and future fertility. Journal of Women's Health (2002). 2003;**12**:513-520

[61] Kaufman FR, Kogut MD, Donnell GN, Goebelsmann U, March C, Koch R. Hypergonadotrophic hypogonadism in female patients with galactosemia. The New England Journal of Medicine. 1981;**304**:994-998

[62] Bjursell C, Stibler H, Wahlström J, et al. Fine mapping of the gene for carbohydrate-deficient glycoprotein syndrome, type 1 (CDG1): Linkage disequilibrium and founder effect in Scandinavian families. Genomics. 1997;**39**:247-253

[63] Yanase T. 17α-hydroxylase/17, 20-lyse defects. The Journal of Steroid Biochemistry and Molecular Biology. 1995;**53**:153-157

[64] Mullis PE, Yoshimura N, Kuhlmann B, Lippuner K, Jaeger P, Harada H. Aromatase deficiency in a female who is compared heterozygote for two new point mutations in the P450arom gene: Impact of estrogens on hypergonadotrophic hypogonadism, multicystic ovaries, and bone densitometry in childhood. The Journal of Clinical Endocrinology and Metabolism. 1997;**82**:1739-1745

[65] Van Dorp W, Mulder RL, Kremer LCM, et al. Recommendations for premature ovarian insufficiency surveillance for female survivors of childhood, adolescent, and young adult cancer: A report from the international Late Effects of Childhood Cancer Guideline Harmonization Group in collaboration with the PanCareSurFupConsortium. Journal of Clinical Oncology. 2016;**34**:3440-3450

[66] Wallace WH. Oncofertility and preservation of reproductive capacity in children and young adults. Cancer. 2011;**117**:2301-2310

[67] Beerendonk CC, Braat DD. Present and future options for the preservation of fertility in female adolescents with cancer. Endocrine Development. 2005;**8**:166-175

[68] Lie Fong S, Laven JS, Hakvoort-Cammel FG, Schipper I, Visser JA, Themmen AP, et al. Assessment of ovarian reserve in adult childhood cancer survivors using anti-Mullerian hormone. Human Reproduction. 2009;**24**:982-990

[69] Wallace WH, Thomson AB, Saran F, Kelsey TW. Predicting age of ovarian failure after radiation to a field that includes the ovaries. International Journal of Radiation Oncology, Biology, Physics. 2005;**62**:738-744

[70] Gracia CR, Sammel MD, Freeman E, Prewitt M, Carlson C, Ray A, et al. Impact of cancer therapies on ovarian reserve. Fertility and Sterility. 2012;**97**:134-140. e131

[71] Siddle N, Sarrel P, Whitehead M. The effect of hysterectomy on the age at ovarian failure: Identification of a subgroup of women with premature loss of ovarian function and literature review. Fertility and Sterility. 1987;**47**:94-100

[72] Visvanathan N, Wyshak G. Tubal ligation, menstrual changes, and menopausal symptoms. Journal of Women's Health & Gender-Based Medicine. 2000;**9**:521-527

[73] Coccia ME, Rizzello F, Mariani G, Bulletti C, Palagiano A, Scarselli G. Ovarian surgery for bilateral endometriomas influences age at menopause. Human Reproduction. 2011;**26**:3000-3007

[74] Fenton A, Panay N. Does routine gynecological surgery contribute to an early menopause? Climacteric. 2012;**15**:1-2

[75] Api M. Is ovarian reserve diminished after laparoscopic ovarian drilling? Gynecological Endocrinology. 2009;**25**:159-165

[76] Koh JM, Kim CH, Hong SK, Lee KU, Kim YT, Kim OJ, et al. Primary ovarian failure caused by a solvent containing 2- bromopropane. European Journal of Endocrinology. 1998;**138**(5):554-556

[77] Kappeler CJ, Hoyer PB. vinylcyclohexene diepoxide: A model chemical for ovotoxicity. Systems Biology in Reproductive Medicine. 2012 Feb;**58**(1):57-62. DOI: 10.3109/19396368.2011.648820. 4

[78] Matkainen T. Aromatic hydrocarbon receptor-driven Bax gene expression. Nature Genetics. 2001;**28**:355-360. DOI: 10.1038/ng575

[79] Kokcu A. Premature ovarian failure from current perspective. Gynecological Endocrinology. 2010;**26**:555-562

[80] Morrison JC, Givens JR, Wiser WL, Fish SA. Mumps oophoritis: A cause of premature menopause. Fertility and Sterility. 1975;**26**:655-659

[81] Imai K, Sutton MY, Mdodo R, Del Rio C. HIV and menopause: A systematic review of the effects of HIV infection of age at menopause and the effects if menopause on response to antiretroviral therapy. Obstetrics and Gynecology International. 2013;**2013**:11. Article ID: 340309. http://dx.doi.org/10.1155/2013/340309

[82] Liao KL, Wood N, Conway GS. Premature menopause and psychological well-being. Journal of Psychosomatic Obstetrics and Gynaecology. 2000;**21**:167-174

[83] International Premature Ovarian Failure Association. Alexandria, VA, USA. Available from: http://www.pofsupport.org [Accessed: August 10, 2013]

[84] Rivera CM, Grossardt B, Rhodes D, et al. Increased cardiovascular mortality after early bilateral oophorectomy. Menopause. 2009;**16**:15-23

[85] Welt CK. Primary ovarian insufficiency: A more accurate term for premature ovarian failure. Clinical Endocrinology. 2009;**68**:449-509. DOI: 10. 1111/j.1365-2265.2007. 03073.x

[86] Rossouw JE, Anderson GL, Prentice RL, LaCroix AZ, Kooperberg C, Stefanick ML, et al. Risks and benefits of estrogen plus progestin in healthy postmenopausal women: Principal results from the women's health initiative randomized controlled trial. JAMA. 2002;**288**:321-333

[87] Mishell DR Jr, Nakamura RM, Crosignani PG, et al. Serum gonadotropin and steroid patterns during the normal menstrual cycle. American Journal of Obstetrics and Gynecology. 1971;**111**(1):60-65

[88] Scarabin PY, Alhenc-Gelas M, Plu-Bureau G, et al. Effects of oral and transdermal estrogen/progesterone regimens on blood coagulation and fibrinolysis in postmenopausal women. A randomized controlled trial. Arteriosclerosis, Thrombosis, and Vascular Biology. 1997;**17**(11):3071-3078

[89] Scarabin PY, Oger E, Plu-Bureau G. Differential association of oral and transdermal oestrogen replacement therapy with venous thromboembolism risk. Lancet. 2003; **362**(9382):428-432

[90] Canonico M, Oger E, Plu-Bureau G, et al. Hormone therapy and venous thromboembolism among postmenopausal women: Impact of the route of estrogen administration and progestogens: The ESTHER study. Circulation. 2007;**115**(7):840-845

[91] Gibbons WE, Moyer DL, Lobo RA, et al. Biochemical and histologic effects of sequential estrogen/progestin therapy on the endometrium of postmenopausal women. American Journal of Obstetrics and Gynecology. 1986;**154**(2):456-461. PubMed: 3004222

[92] Davis SR, Burger HG. The role of androgen therapy. Best Practice & Research. Clinical Endocrinology & Metabolism. 2003;**17**:165-175

[93] Arlt W. Androgen therapy in women. European Journal of Endocrinology. 2006;**154**:1-11

[94] Ankarberg-Lindgren C, Elfving M, Wikland KA, Norjavaara E. Nocturnal application of transdermal estradiol patches produces levels of estradiol that mimic those seen at the onset of spontaneous puberty in girls. The Journal of Clinical Endocrinology and Metabolism. 2001;**86**:3039-3044

[95] Davenport ML. Approach to the patient with Turner syndrome. The Journal of Clinical Endocrinology and Metabolism. 2010;**95**:1487-1495

[96] Schenck-Gustaffson K, Brincat M, Erel T, Gambacciani M, Lamberdounaki I, Tremorrlieres F, et al. EMAS position statement: Managing the menopause in the context of coronary heart disease. Maturitas. 2011;**68**:94-97

[97] Beljic T, Zivkovic T, Vuksanovic M, Andjelic-Jelic M, Stojanovic J, Buric B, et al. Obesity and metabolic syndrome during the menopausal transition. Climacteric. 2011;**14**:643-648

[98] Shuster LT, Rhodes DJ, Gostout BS, Grossardt BR, Rocca WA. Premature menopause or early menopause: Long-term health consequences. Maturitas. 2010;**65**:161-166

[99] Kannel WB, Hjortland MC, McNamara PM, Gordon T. Menopause and risk of cardiovascular disease. The Framingham study. Annals of Internal Medicine. 1976;**85**:447-452

[100] Faubion SS, Kuhle CL, Shuster LT, Rocca WA. Long-term health consequences of premature or early menopause and considerations for management. Climacteric. 2015;**18**:483-491

[101] Popat VB, Calis KA, Vanderhoof VH, Cizza G, Reynolds JC, Sebring N, et al. Bone mineral density in estrogen-deficient young women. The Journal of Clinical Endocrinology and Metabolism. 2009;**94**(7):2277-2283

[102] Vega EM, Egea MA, Mautalen CA. Influence of the menopausal age on the severity of osteoporosis in women with vertebral fractures. Maturitas. 1994;**19**:117-124

[103] Van der Klift M, de Laet CE, McCloskey EV, et al. Risk factors for incident vertebral fractures in men and women: The Rotterdam study. Journal of Bone and Mineral Research. 2004;**19**:1172-1180

[104] Rocca WA, Bower JH, Maraganore DM, et al. Increased risk of parkinsonism in women who underwent oophorectomy before menopause. Neurology. 2009;**70**:200-209

[105] Rocca WA, Bower JH, Maraganore DM, et al. Increased risk of cognitive impairment or dementia in women who underwent oophorectomy before menopause. Neurology. 2007;**69**:1074-1083

[106] Phung TK, Waltoft BL, Laursen TM, et al. Hysterectomy, oophorectomy and risk of dementia: A nationwide historical cohort study. Dementia and Geriatric Cognitive Disorders. 2010;**30**:43-50

[107] Nelson LM, Covington SN, Rebar RW. An update: Spontaneous premature ovarian failure is not an early menopause. Fertility and Sterility. 2005;**83**:1327-1332

[108] Nelson LM, Anasti JN, Kimzey LM, et al. Development of luteinized graafian follicles in patients with karyotypically normal spontaneous premature ovarian failure. The Journal of Clinical Endocrinology and Metabolism. 1994 Nov;**79**(5):1470-1475

[109] Taylor AE, Adams JM, Mulder JE, Martin KA, Sluss PM, Crowley WF,J. A randomized, controlled trial of estradiol replacement therapy in women with hypergonadotrophic amenorrhea. The Journal of Clinical Endocrinology and Metabolism. 1996;**81**:3615-3621

[110] Tartagni M, Cicinelli E, De Pergola G, et al. Effects of pretreatment with estrogens on ovarian stimulation with gonadotropins in women with premature ovarian failure: A randomized, placebo-controlled trial. Fertility and Sterility. 2007;**87**:858-861

[111] Mamas L, Mamas E. Premature ovarian failure and dehydroepiandrosterone. Fertility and Sterility. 2009;**91**:644-646

[112] Badawy A, Goda H, Ragab A. Induction of ovulation in idiopathic premature ovarian failure: A randomized double-blind trial. Reproductive Biomedicine Online. 2007;**15**:215-219

[113] Ferrau F, Gangemi S, Vita G, Trimarchi F, Cannavo S. Pregnancy after azathioprine therapy for ulcerative colitis in a woman with autoimmune premature ovarian failure and Addison's disease: HLA haplotype characterization. Fertility and Sterility. 2011;**95**:2430 e2415-2430 e2437

[114] Sauer MV, Paulson RJ, Ary BA, Lobo RA. Three hundred cycles of oocyte donation at the University of Southern California: Assessing the effect of age and infertility diagnosis on pregnancy and implantation rates. Journal of Assisted Reproduction and Genetics. 1994;**11**:92-96

[115] Templeton A, Morris JK, Parslow W. Factors that affect outcome of in-vitro fertilisation treatment. Lancet. 1996;**348**:1402-1406

[116] Foudila T, Soderstrom-Antilla V, Hovatta O. Turner's syndrome and pregnancies after oocyte donation. Human Reproduction. 1999;**14**:532-535

[117] Practice Committee of the American Society for Reproductive Medicine. Increased maternal cardiovascular mortality associated with pregnancy in women with Turner syndrome. Fertility and Sterility. 2012 Feb;**97**(2):0015-0282. DOI: 10.1016/j.fertnstert.2011.11.049

[118] Michala L, Goswami D, Creighton SM, Conway GS. Swyer syndrome: Presentation and outcomes. BJOG. 2008;**115**:737-741

[119] Rocha VB, Guerra-Júnior G, Marques-de-Faria AP, de Mello MP, Maciel-Guerra AT. Complete gonadal dysgenesis in clinical practice: The 46, XY karyotype accounts for more than one third of cases. Fertility and Sterility. 2011 Dec;**96**(6):1431-1434. DOI: 10.1016/j.fertnstert.2011.09.009. Epub 2011 Oct 6

[120] Wong KM, Mastenbroek S, Repping S. Cryopreservation of human embryos and it contribution to *in vitro* fertilization success rates. Fertility and Sterility. 2014;**102**:19-26

[121] Evans J, Hannan NJ, Edgell TA, et al. Fresh versus frozen embryo transfer: Backing clinical decisions with scientific and clinical evidence. Human Reproduction Update. 2014;**20**:808-821

[122] Grifo JA, Noyes N. Delivery rate using cryopreserved oocytes is comparable to conventional *in vitro* fertilization using fresh oocytes: Potential fertility preservation for female cancer patients. Fertility and Sterility. 2010;**93**:391-396

[123] Oktay K, Karlikaya G. Ovarian function after transplantation of frozen, banked autologous ovarian tissue. The New England Journal of Medicine. 2000;**342**:1919

[124] Donnez J, Silber S, Andersen CY. Children born after autotransplantation of cryopreserved ovarian tissue: A review of 13 live births. Annals of Medicine. 2011;**43**:437-450

[125] Schmidt KT, Resendahl M, Ernst E. Autotransplantation of cryopreserved ovarian tissue in 12 women with chemotherapy-induced premature ovarian failure: The Danish experience. Fertility and Sterility. 2011;**95**:695-701

[126] Conway GS, Payne NN, Webb J, Murray A, Jacobs PA. Fragile X premutation screening in women with premature ovarian failure. Human Reproduction. 1998;**13**:1184-1187

[127] Vegetti W, Grazia Tibiletti M, Testa G, de Lauretis Y, Alagna F, Castoldi E, et al. Inheritance in idiopathic premature ovarian failure: Analysis of 71 cases. Human Reproduction. 1998;**13**:1796-1800

[128] van Kasteren YM, Hundscheid RD, Smits AP, Cremers FP, van Zonneveld P, Braat DD. Familial idiopathic premature ovarian failure: An overrated and underestimated genetic disease? Human Reproduction. 1999;**14**:2455-2459

[129] Janse F, Knauff EA, Niermeijer MF, Eijkemans MJ, Laven JS, Lambalk CB, et al. Dutch Premature Ovarian Failure C. Similar phenotype characteristics comparing familial and sporadic premature ovarian failure. Menopause. 2010;**17**:758-765

[130] McConkie-Rosell A, Finucane B, Cronister A, Abrams L, Bennett RL, Pettersen BJ. Genetic counseling for fragile x syndrome: Updated recommendations of the national society of genetic counselors. Journal of Genetic Counseling. 2005;**14**:249-270

[131] Dunlop CE, Telfer EE, Anderson RA. Ovarian stem cells--potential roles in infertility treatment and fertility preservation. Maturitas. 2013 Nov;**76**(3):279-283. DOI: 10.1016/j.maturitas.2013.04.017. Epub 2013 May 18

[132] Kawamura K, Cheng Y, Suzuki N, Deguchi M, Sato Y, Takae S, et al. Hippo signaling disruption and Akt stimulation of ovarian follicles for infertility treatment. Proceedings of the National Academy of Sciences of the United States of America. 2013 Oct 22;**110**(43):17474-17479. DOI: 10.1073/pnas.1312830110

[133] Zhai J, Yao G, Dong F, Bu Z, Cheng Y, Sato Y, et al. In vitro activation of follicles and fresh tissue auto-transplantation in primary ovarian insufficiency patients. The Journal of Clinical Endocrinology & Metabolism. 2016 Nov 1;**101**(11):4405-4412. DOI: 10.1210/jc.2016-158

Chapter 7

# Standardization of Menstrual Cycle Data for the Analysis of Intensive Longitudinal Data

Kayla M. Joyce and Sherry H. Stewart

Additional information is available at the end of the chapter

http://dx.doi.org/10.5772/intechopen.81504

**Abstract**

Daily diary methodology is becoming popular in human menstrual cycle (MC) research. However, variations in MC length makes it difficult to examine fluctuations in dependent variables (e.g., substance use levels), across the MC. Existing analytic approaches collapse data across MC phases, examining phase-related changes; however, a loss of potentially vital information can result when data is collapsed across phase. Additionally, current phase designation methods (phase designation and days within each phase) vary substantially across studies, making it difficult to interpret/compare results across studies. To address these problems, two methods were developed to standardize intensive longitudinal data collected via daily diary methodologies—phasic and continuous standardization. Phasic standardization accounts for individual variability in MC length by allowing luteal phase length differences while remaining phases are fixed, enabling the analysis of phasic variations. Alternatively, continuous standardization accounts for individual variability in MC length by standardizing the luteal phase to a seven-day phase, while remaining phases are fixed, allowing for the exploration of continuously reported variables across MC day. This chapter will discuss how to standardize daily diary data collected across the MC using phasic and continuous standardization methods and demonstrate the two standardization methods using two clinically-relevant hypothetical examples.

**Keywords:** addiction, substance use, behavioral addiction, mood, menstrual cycle

## 1. Introduction

Historically, females have been omitted from addictions research. One reason for this omission is that ovarian hormones fluctuate rhythmically across females' menstrual cycles and may impact their addictive behavior. As a result of this sex bias, theory and evidence pertaining to the nature, development, and maintenance of addiction are based primarily on research with male samples [1]. Given that females have been underrepresented in addictions research, many treatment and preventative intervention methods developed to date may not be suitable for females with addictions. This general failure to develop sex-specific treatment and prevention options is particularly problematic given the high occurrence of addictive behaviors in females. For example, the National Council on Alcoholism and Drug Dependence [2] has reported that 4.5 million American females abuse/are dependent on alcohol, 3.5 million misuse prescription drugs, and 3.1 million regularly use illicit drugs. Of further concern, the Substance Abuse and Mental Health Services Administration [3] has reported that 15.8 million American females, 18 years and older, have used illicit drugs within the past year. These statistics exemplify just how common addictive behaviors are in the female population.

Of further concern, the prevalence of addictive behaviors in females is increasing and closely approaching that of men. For example, increases in females' alcohol consumption and alcohol use disorders are evident, with prevalence rates converging upon those reported for males [4]. The documented convergence between female and male alcohol consumption and alcohol use disorders may be explained by a societal shift toward an increased acceptance for females to engage in potentially addictive behaviors, such as alcohol consumption and tobacco use [5]. Thus, investigating sex-specific factors influencing addictive behaviors is critical for the development of effective treatment and prevention options for females with addictions.

As a result of the current underrepresentation of females in addiction research and our substandard knowledge of sex-specific factors influencing addiction, many funding agencies (e.g., Canadian Institute of Health Research) have introduced a requirement that researchers consider sex when developing research questions and designs. With this sex-sensitive research focus, numerous researchers have begun exploring the potential influence of the menstrual cycle, a female-specific factor, on fluctuations in addictive behaviors (e.g., cigarettes smoked, gambling intensity) and mood (e.g., negative and positive affect).

To effectively examine fluctuations in addictive behavior across the menstrual cycle, researchers have begun employing daily diaries—a prospective methodology where participants are asked to complete surveys at various time points throughout the day. Using daily diary surveys provides researchers with the advantage of obtaining intensive longitudinal data. However, variation in female menstrual cycle length has made it particularly difficult to conduct such daily diary menstrual cycle research due to the lack of established menstrual cycle standardization methodologies. Since researchers currently do not have a method to standardize variable menstrual cycle lengths, they are left with the sole option of breaking the menstrual cycle down into phases which vary not only in length across studies but also by the total number of menstrual cycle phases, which can be problematic.

Currently, two predominant problems in menstrual cycle research are evident. First is the lack of comparability across studies with respect to the data which goes into each menstrual cycle phase. Although the division of data into menstrual cycle phases itself is not necessarily problematic, issues appear when inconsistencies arise within phase designation methods across studies. Researchers commonly divide the menstrual cycle into a different number of menstrual cycle phases, with each phase consisting of various days, which further confounds the picture. Inconsistencies in menstrual cycle phase designations were demonstrated in a literature review where studies reporting addictive behaviors across the menstrual cycle were examined. In our literature review, two studies, both examining sexual behavior across menstrual cycle phase, divided the menstrual cycle into two and seven menstrual cycle phases, respectively [6, 7]. Two additional studies, examining cigarette use/nicotine intake across the menstrual cycle, designated the premenstrual phase as 3 and 5 days prior to menstruation, respectively [8, 9]. With these evident discrepancies in menstrual cycle phase designation between studies, our ability to effectively compare research findings is substantially limited. To effectively compare research findings in the menstrual cycle field, the development of standardization methods is warranted. Given these problems, we propose a method to standardize menstrual cycle phase given variable menstrual cycle lengths across different female participants. Throughout this book chapter we will refer to this form of standardization as 'phasic standardization' which can be analyzed using statistical methods such as repeated-measures analyses of variance (ANOVAs), for example.

Even though phasic standardization eliminates one problem, another problem arises. When data is collapsed across days within phases, a daily average per phase is produced. However, collapsing data across menstrual cycle phase to produce a phasic average still results in a loss of potentially important information. Instead, data can be examined continuously across menstrual cycle days using another form of standardization to eliminate the problem of collapsing data across days within each menstrual cycle phase. As a solution to this second problem, we propose a method to standardize menstrual cycle day given variable menstrual cycle lengths across females. Throughout, we refer to this as 'continuous standardization'[1], which can be analyzed using data analytic techniques like time varying effects models (TVEMs).

The current chapter aims to eliminate the standardization problem in menstrual cycle research by providing a method for researchers to standardize intensive longitudinal data collected using daily diary methodology across the female menstrual cycle. We will explain how researchers can standardize such intensive longitudinal data across the menstrual cycle using one of two methods (i.e., phasic or continuous standardization). We also provide two clinically-relevant hypothetical examples of the proposed standardization methods. We will also explore the statistical methods which can be used to analyze such standardized menstrual cycle data, including repeated measures ANOVAs and TVEMs. This book chapter may be of practical use to researchers working in the menstrual cycle field as it provides standardized methodology for examining fluctuations in dependent variables, such as substance use levels and mood, across the menstrual cycle. The purpose of this chapter is to provide standardization methods to examine menstrual cycle data as means to enhance our understanding of the menstrual cycle as a female-specific factor in the field of addiction and mental health.

[1]Please note that continuous standardization does not refer to the continuous nature of the dependent variable or continuous outcomes but rather examining data at the daily level (continuously) rather than at the phasic level.

## 2. Menstrual cycle data standardization

On average, a female's menstrual cycle lasts between 23 and 35 days (average length = 28 days) [10], indicating a large range of individual variability in menstrual cycle length. Based on ovarian hormone fluctuations, the menstrual cycle has been divided into two overarching phases: the follicular (from menstrual bleeding until ovulation) and luteal phases (from ovulation until the day prior to menstrual bleeding) [11]. Furthermore, rhythmic fluctuations in progesterone, estrogen, follicle-stimulating hormone, and luteinizing hormone concentrations, allow for further subdivision of the menstrual cycle, resulting in the following five more specific phases: menstrual, follicular, ovulatory, luteal, and premenstrual [11–14] (see **Figure 1**).

Variability in female menstrual cycle length has been attributed to differing luteal phase lengths [15]. Although the literature is mixed in the sense that some literature points toward the follicular phase as the phase that contributes the most to menstrual cycle variability [16], the bulk of the literature suggests that the luteal phase is the main contributor to variance in menstrual cycle length [15]. That menstrual cycle length variability occurs specifically at the luteal phase is supported by two facts. Firstly, although the timing of the ovulatory phase may differ on an individual basis, research shows the ovulatory phase typically occurs between days 13–16 of the menstrual cycle [11] suggesting there is little variability prior to the ovulatory phase. The second is that the premenstrual phase has been defined as occurring 5 days prior to menstrual bleeding [17]. Thus, it is the luteal phase, which precedes the menstrual phase, that is subject to variable lengths. Based on the fact that variability in a female's menstrual cycle occurs during the luteal phase, we have developed two methods to standardize menstrual cycle data, consisting of phasic and continuous standardization, respectively (see Sections 2 and 3 for methodological procedures and clinically-relevant hypothetical

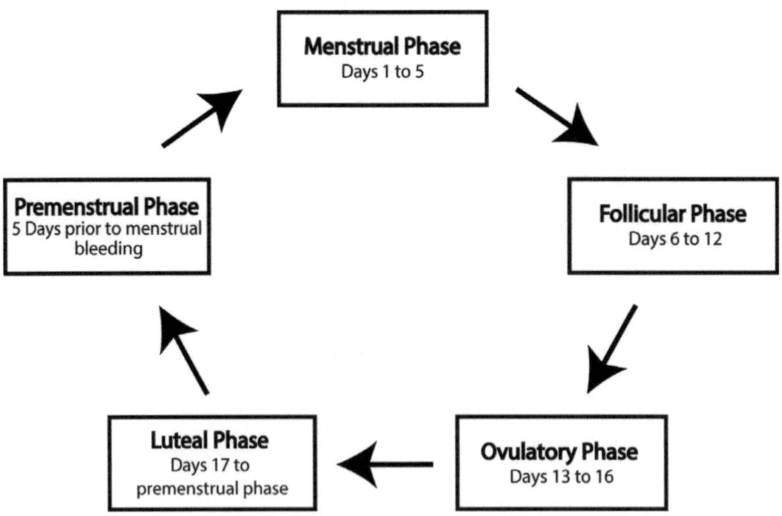


**Figure 1.** A depiction of the menstrual cycle divided into five specific phases.

examples of the two standardization methods). It is cautioned that the two standardization methods described herein solely be implemented for menstrual cycle lengths between 23 and 35 days. Females with menstrual cycle lengths outside of the average 23–35 days should not be included in the menstrual cycle standardization methods discussed in this chapter. The accuracy of standardizing data from females with menstrual cycle lengths outside of the average 23- to 35-day range is questionable. Abnormally short/long menstrual cycles have an unduly influential role in ovarian hormone fluctuations. Thus, such individuals are typically categorized as not normally-cycling and are not included in studies of the normal female menstrual cycle [10].

### 2.1. Phasic standardization

If a researcher is interested in variations in specific behaviors (e.g., substance use or other addictive behavior) occurring during certain phases of the menstrual cycle, we have developed a standardized method to examine phase-related changes in behavior. We refer to this standardization method as phasic standardization. In this method, data collected via daily diary across an entire menstrual cycle is standardized as a means for examining addictive behaviors by phase rather than as a function of days across the entire menstrual cycle (see continuous standardization in the next section of the chapter). When conducting phasic standardization, all menstrual cycle phases are held at fixed lengths, save the length of the luteal phase which will differ based on the participant's total menstrual cycle length. Each phase length is as follows: menstrual (days 1–5), follicular (days 6–12), ovulatory (days 13–16), luteal (days 17-premenstrual phase), and premenstrual (5 days prior to menstrual bleeding; see **Table 1**). Each variable of interest is examined as a mean per phase. Each mean per phase variable is calculated by summing each variable per phase and dividing that sum by the total number of days within that menstrual cycle phase.

Data obtained through phasic standardization can be analyzed through the implementation of statistical methods such as repeated-measures ANOVAs or dependent-sample planned contrasts. A repeated-measures ANOVA will identify whether there is a significant difference across menstrual cycle phases on a given dependent variable (e.g., bidding quantity). If the repeated-measures ANOVA reveals a significant effect of MC phase, post-hoc comparisons can be conducted to determine which menstrual cycle phase(s) are characterized by higher/lower levels of the dependent variable relative to which other MC phase(s).

### 2.2. Continuous standardization

Since variability in menstrual cycle length occurs during the luteal phase [15], the luteal phase can be standardized to a seven-day phase, based on the average 28-day cycle, while the remaining phases are held fixed. We refer to this method as continuous standardization. Upon conducting continuous standardization, the length at which each phase is held constant is as follows: 5 days for the menstrual phase (menstrual cycle days 1–5), 7 days for the follicular phase (menstrual cycle days 6–12), 4 days for the ovulatory phase (menstrual cycle days 13–16), and 5 days for the premenstrual phase (5 days prior to menstrual bleeding), accumulating to a total of 21 days. Next, the 21 days are subtracted from the participant's total menstrual cycle

| Menstrual cycle day | Menstrual cycle phase | Bidding occasions | Average number of bidding occasions per phase |
|---|---|---|---|
| 1 | | 8 | |
| 2 | | 6 | |
| 3 | Menstrual | 0 | 4 |
| 4 | | 2 | |
| 5 | | 4 | |
| 6 | | 11 | |
| 7 | | 2 | |
| 8 | | 8 | |
| 9 | Follicular | 10 | 6 |
| 10 | | 6 | |
| 11 | | 0 | |
| 12 | | 5 | |
| 13 | | 13 | |
| 14 | Ovulatory | 8 | 9 |
| 15 | | 7 | |
| 16 | | 8 | |
| 17 | Luteal | 8 | 7 |
| 18 | | 6 | |
| 19 | | 2 | |
| 20 | | 1 | |
| 21 | Premenstrual | 4 | 2 |
| 22 | | 0 | |
| 23 | | 3 | |

**Table 1.** Method to standardize intensive longitudinal data into the five menstrual cycle phases using phasic standardization.

length. The remainder provides the total number of days in the participant's luteal phase (see **Table 2**). All participant's menstrual cycles can then be standardized to a 28-day cycle by allotting 7 standardized days to the participant's luteal phase length (i.e., 28-day cycle – 21 days (sum of non-luteal phase days) = 7-day luteal phase). Thus, we can express the variance as a ratio of 7/x where x is the participant's actual luteal phase length (see **Table 2**). With this luteal phase ratio, we can determine the standardized luteal phase day for each actual luteal phase day. This is calculated by treating the ratio as a factor to be added to day 16 (the last day of the ovulatory phase) to obtain the standardized luteal phase day (see **Table 2**). Each number obtained is then rounded up (≥0.5) or down (<0.5) to the nearest whole number, representing the new standardized luteal phase day. This method can be used for menstrual cycle lengths shorter and longer than the average 28-day cycle. For cycle lengths shorter than 28 days, data from the luteal phase will be "elongated", and data will be missing for certain menstrual cycle days during the luteal phase. Conversely, for cycle lengths longer than 28 days, data from the luteal phase will be "condensed", and the same standardized day may be obtained for two data points (i.e., two data points may be identified as standardized luteal phase day 18). In the latter circumstance, any variables of interest with the same standardized luteal phase day must be averaged and that datapoint will be linked to the given standardized luteal phase day.

Menstrual cycle data standardized using continuous standardization can be analyzed using more intricate statistical analyses, such as TVEMs [18]. TVEMs allow for the identification

| Total menstrual cycle length | Luteal phase length[a] | Luteal phase ratio[b] | Standardized menstrual cycle day[c] |
|---|---|---|---|
| 23 days | 2 | 7/2 | 3.5 |
| 24 days | 3 | 7/3 | $2.\overline{33}$ |
| 25 days | 4 | 7/4 | 1.75 |
| 26 days | 5 | 7/5 | 1.4 |
| 27 days | 6 | 7/6 | $1.1\overline{6}$ |
| 28 days | 7 | 7/7 | 1 |
| 29 days | 8 | 7/8 | .875 |
| 30 days | 9 | 7/9 | $.\overline{77}$ |
| 31 days | 10 | 7/10 | .70 |
| 32 days | 11 | 7/11 | $.6\overline{36}$ |
| 33 days | 12 | 7/12 | $.58\overline{3}$ |
| 34 days | 13 | 7/13 | .538 |
| 35 days | 14 | 7/14 | .50 |

**Table 2.** Method to standardize continuous intensive longitudinal data to a 28-day menstrual cycle.

of cyclical changes in addictive behaviors, mood, and their inter-relations as a function of menstrual cycle day by providing an estimate of the relationship between predictor and outcome variables. TVEMs can function similarly to a mediational analysis over time as they identify menstrual cycle days on which elevations (or reductions) in an outcome variable are due to elevations (or reductions) in another variable. For example, in our prior research we used TVEMs to demonstrate that elevations in alcohol consumption during days corresponding to the menstrual phase were explained by elevations in coping drinking motives during these same menstrual cycle days. The implementation of such statistical analyses allows for a more comprehensive understanding of the relationship between addictive behaviors and other factors.

In our prior research [19], we have biologically validated standardizing menstrual cycle length via continuous standardization through the collection of saliva samples. In our research, we collected saliva samples during times of theoretically low (days 1–7) and high (days 18–24) progesterone concentrations [19]. Enzyme-linked immunosorbent assays (ELISA) were then carried out to determine progesterone concentrations for each participant and a paired-sample t-test followed to validate participant's menstrual cycle day using the identified progesterone concentrations. Results suggested that menstrual cycle days 18–24 (theoretical high) had significantly higher progesterone concentrations than menstrual cycle days 1–7 (theoretical low). Findings provided biological validation for standardizing menstrual cycle data via continuous standardization based on an average 28-day menstrual cycle.

## 3. Clinically-relevant examples

To provide a more comprehensive understanding of the methods employed to standardize data, we have developed two clinically-relevant hypothetical examples. These hypothetical examples were designed to illustrate the types of effects that have been established in the literature on addictive behaviors across the menstrual cycle.

### 3.1. Phasic example: gambling involvement

In this hypothetical example, the researchers wanted to examine bidding quantity per menstrual cycle phase to determine if bidding quantity increases or decreases during specific phases of the menstrual cycle relative to other phases of the menstrual cycle (e.g., does bidding frequency increase during the ovulatory phase relative to other menstrual cycle phases?). Let us imagine that this hypothetical data was collected using daily diary methodology. Each day for an entire menstrual cycle, female gambler participants were asked to report their menstrual cycle day and the number of times they bid throughout the day. Here, the researchers collapsed the data by phase, using phasic standardization, to assess whether differences in bidding frequency occurred as a function of menstrual cycle phase.

Using the phasic standardization method, we can produce standardized data that allows for the comparison of data at specific menstrual cycle phases between participants, even though such phases may not be identical in length (see **Figure 2** for a hypothetical example). Phasic standardization is conducted in the same manner, regardless of the participant's menstrual cycle length. Collectively, using phasic standardization allows for the identification of phase-specific differences in addictive behaviors (or mood states, for example) across the menstrual cycle.

Phasic standardization can be illustrated with a hypothetical example (see **Table 3**). Here the fictional participant's 23-day menstrual cycle can be divided into five menstrual cycle phases as outlined in Section 2.1 above. In **Table 3**, the luteal phase is comprised of all days that are not non-luteal phase days (i.e., days that are not accounted for by another menstrual cycle phase where the other phases are of fixed length). In this hypothetical example, days 17–18 represent the luteal phase. Once the data is divided based on menstrual cycle phase, the bidding quantity variable was averaged for all days within each specific phase. Using phasic

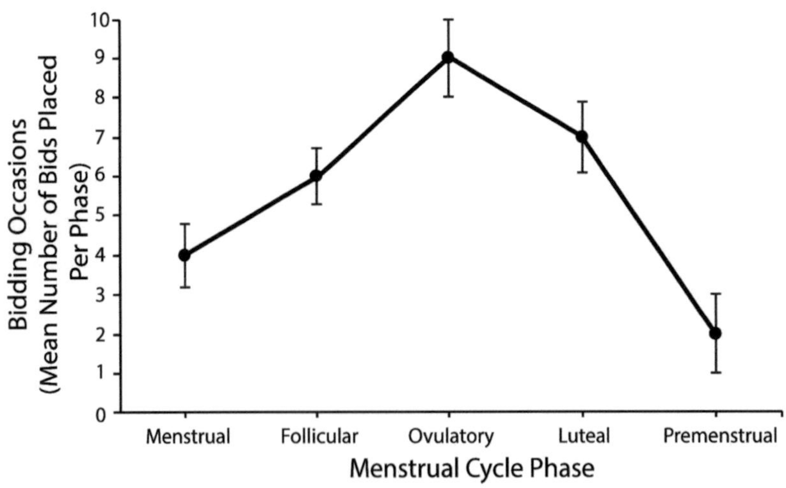


**Figure 2.** Example of the mean number of bidding occasions across the five menstrual cycle phases. Error bars represent standard error.

http://dx.doi.org/10.5772/intechopen.81504

standardization, we obtain one datapoint for each variable of interest per phase per participant. Based on the hypothetical case discussed (see **Table 3**), it appears as though the average number of bidding occasions is lowest during the menstrual phase, peaks during the ovulatory phase, and progressively declines thereafter, consistent with the researcher's hypothesis. Once collapsed across participants in the sample, these phasic means can be compared using statistics like repeated-measures ANOVA to answer the researcher's question of whether bidding increases during the ovulatory phase relative to the other menstrual cycle phases.

### 3.2. Continuous example: cigarettes smoked

In this second hypothetical example, imagine that a group of researchers wanted to examine cigarette use across the entire menstrual cycle (i.e., across days) to elucidate if, and where, cigarette use increases or decreases across the menstrual cycle. Imagine that these researchers collected information using daily diary surveys to determine participant menstrual cycle day and the number of cigarettes smoked each day across each participant's entire menstrual cycle. Let us imagine that the researchers in this example were primarily interested in examining cigarette use across the entirety of the menstrual cycle to determine where the level of cigarettes smoked rise and fall (i.e., which menstrual cycle days). This more specific level of

| Menstrual cycle day | Menstrual cycle phase | Bidding occasions | Average number of bidding occasions per phase |
|---|---|---|---|
| 1 | | 8 | |
| 2 | | 6 | |
| 3 | Menstrual | 0 | 4 |
| 4 | | 2 | |
| 5 | | 4 | |
| 6 | | 11 | |
| 7 | | 2 | |
| 8 | | 8 | |
| 9 | Follicular | 10 | 6 |
| 10 | | 6 | |
| 11 | | 0 | |
| 12 | | 5 | |
| 13 | | 13 | |
| 14 | Ovulatory | 8 | 9 |
| 15 | | 7 | |
| 16 | | 8 | |
| 17 | Luteal | 8 | 7 |
| 18 | | 6 | |
| 19 | | 2 | |
| 20 | | 1 | |
| 21 | Premenstrual | 4 | 2 |
| 22 | | 0 | |
| 23 | | 3 | |

**Table 3.** A worked hypothetical example of the phasic method for standardizing a 23-day menstrual cycle across the five phases.

detail might not be captured using a phasic evaluation; thus, these researchers would choose to employ continuous standardization rather than phasic standardization.

As mentioned previously, in a normally-cycling sample, we would expect inclusion of individuals who have menstrual cycle lengths that are below and others who have menstrual cycle lengths that are above the average menstrual cycle length of 28 days. Given this, we will provide two examples of continuous standardization using each of these types of cases (i.e., longer than average cycle lengths, shorter than average cycle lengths, respectively) from a hypothetical dataset.

Using this method, we can produce standardized data with all participants having exactly a 28-day standard menstrual cycle (see **Figure 3** for an example). This enables us to compare data between participants with variable cycle lengths to determine if specific standardized days are associated with greater (or reduced) addictive behaviors as, following standardization, each day would represent the same time point across participants. Additionally, this process enables us to not only examine specific days, but also identify specific menstrual cycle phases where changes are occurring as all participants have a standardized 28-day cycle with each phase length being consistent across participants. Collectively, we can identify phase-specific and day-specific differences in addictive behaviors across the entirety of the menstrual cycle, using this method of standardization.

### *3.2.1. For cycle lengths fewer than 28 days*

In Section 2.2., we described that the first step in continuous standardization is to calculate the number of luteal phase days by holding all other menstrual cycle phases constant in length. In **Figure 4**, the number of menstrual cycle days is listed for the average 28-day cycle. This information is then utilized to calculate the number of luteal phase days by subtracting the

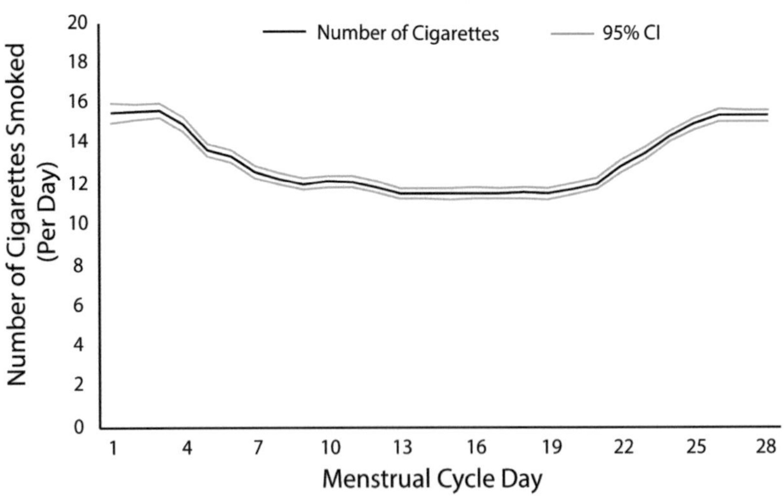


**Figure 3.** Hypothetical example of the mean number of cigarettes smoked across days of the menstrual cycle. Black lines indicate means and gray lines indicate 95% confidence intervals.

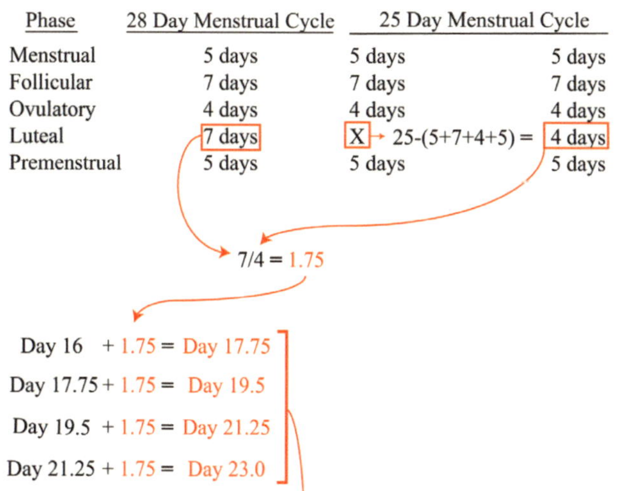


| Menstrual cycle day | Number of cigarettes smoked per day | Standardized menstrual cycle day | *Rounded*: standardized menstrual cycle day | *Standardized Data*: number of cigarettes smoked per day |
|---|---|---|---|---|
| 1 | 16 | 1 | 1 | 16 |
| 2 | 16 | 2 | 2 | 16 |
| 3 | 15 | 3 | 3 | 15 |
| 4 | 15 | 4 | 4 | 15 |
| 5 | 14 | 5 | 5 | 14 |
| 6 | 13 | 6 | 6 | 13 |
| 7 | 12 | 7 | 7 | 12 |
| 8 | 12 | 8 | 8 | 12 |
| 9 | 12 | 9 | 9 | 12 |
| 10 | 12 | 10 | 10 | 12 |
| 11 | 12 | 11 | 11 | 12 |
| 12 | 12 | 12 | 12 | 12 |
| 13 | 12 | 13 | 13 | 12 |
| 14 | 12 | 14 | 14 | 12 |
| 15 | 12 | 15 | 15 | 12 |
| 16 | 12 | 16 | 16 | 12 |
| Luteal Phase 17 | **12** | 17.75 | 17 | — |
| 18 | **12** | 19.50 | 18 | **12** |
| 19 | **12** | 21.25 | 19 | — |
| 20 | **13** | 23 | 20 | **12** |
| 21 | 15 | 24 | 21 | **12** |
| 22 | 15 | 25 | 22 | — |
| 23 | 15 | 26 | 23 | **13** |
| 24 | 15 | 27 | 24 | 15 |
| 25 | 15 | 28 | 25 | 15 |
| | | | 26 | 15 |
| | | | 27 | 15 |
| | | | 28 | 15 |

**Figure 4.** A worked hypothetical example of continuous standardization for a menstrual cycle less than 28-days (i.e., 25-day cycle). Note: A dash (–) signifies a missing data point.

total number of non-luteal phase days from the participant's entire menstrual cycle length. For instance, **Figure 4** illustrates this by subtracting 21 days (non-luteal phase days) from this hypothetical participant's entire 25-day menstrual cycle. The remainder (4 days) then becomes the divisor for the number of luteal phase days within the average 28-day cycle (i.e., seven) to identify the factor that must be successively added to day 16. This adding to day 16 occurs four times in this case (the same value as the number of days within the participant's non-standardized luteal phase) to determine the participant's new standardized luteal phase days. Following the arrows in **Figure 4**, we derive four new standardized luteal phase days, which are then rounded to the nearest whole number and incorporated into our dataset.

The table in **Figure 4** highlights days 17–20 (column one)—the four non-standardized luteal phase days for this hypothetical participant—and the number of cigarettes she smoked on each of these days (column two). Each of the four standardized luteal phase days are then rounded to the nearest whole number (column three). It should be noted that standardizing a cycle with fewer than 28 days to a 28-day cycle will yield a standardized luteal phase with missing data (see resultant standardized dataset in column five of **Figure 4**). By comparing the red boxes between columns two and five, we can see that the data from the 25-day cycle is carried forward into the 'standardized data' column. The resulting data set includes data for this hypothetical participant's standardized 28-day menstrual cycle. The hypothetical participant's data (see **Figure 4**) suggests that cigarette smoking peaks during standardized days 1–5 (i.e., during the menstrual phase) and standardized days 24–28 (i.e., during the premenstrual phase) with a dip mid-cycle (i.e., during the follicular, ovulatory, and luteal phases). To determine where cigarette smoking increases and decreases, the standardized 28-day menstrual cycle can be examined across a larger sample of participants with 28-day standardized cycles using a statistical analysis such as TVEMs.

### *3.2.2. For cycle lengths above 28 days*

The process of standardizing a cycle length above 28-days is similar to that employed for cycle lengths less than 28-days (see **Figure 5**). Using the same hypothetical dataset as an example, we have depicted the standardization method for a second hypothetical participant, this time with a menstrual cycle length of 30 days. When standardizing menstrual cycle data for individuals with cycle lengths greater than 28 days, note that a calculated standardized day may round to the same standardized day as an adjacent day, yielding two data points with identical standardized luteal phase days. In this situation, the data from the identical standardized luteal phase days must be averaged and linked to that standardized luteal phase day. In **Figure 5**, we see that in column three, two red arrows converge upon standardized luteal phase day 18, for example. Thus, on standardized day 18, the number of cigarettes smoked is averaged from the data for the original days 18 and 19 (i.e., $12 + 14/2 = 13$). Then, the new datapoint of 13 is placed into column five to represent standardized data for standardized day 18 for the participant's standardized 28-day menstrual cycle. A similar process is used for obtaining the cigarettes smoked value for standardized day 21 (see **Figure 5**). Consistent with the findings for the hypothetical participant in Section 3.2.1., data from this hypothetical participant (see **Figure 5**) also suggests that cigarette smoking peaks during standardized days 1–5 (i.e., corresponding to the menstrual phase) and standardized days 24–28 (i.e., corresponding to the premenstrual phase) with a dip mid-cycle (i.e., corresponding to the follicular, ovulatory, and luteal phases). Using a larger sample of participants with 28-day standardized cycles, the researchers could employ TVEMs to statistically determine which menstrual cycle days and corresponding phases are associated with increases and decreases in cigarette smoking across a female's menstrual cycle.

One might similarly standardize data on mood across the menstrual cycle, for example, for these same participants. One could then determine whether elevations in negative mood menstrually and premenstrually, for example, account for rises in cigarette smoking on days corresponding to these same phases, again using TVEMs (e.g., see [19]).

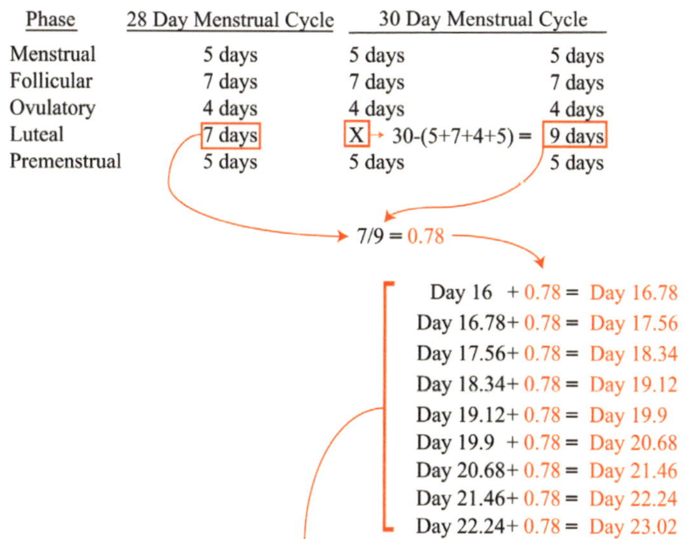


| | Menstrual cycle day | Number of cigarettes smoked per day | Standardized menstrual cycle day | *Rounded*: standardized menstrual cycle day | *Standardized Data*: number of cigarettes smoked per day |
|---|---|---|---|---|---|
| | 1 | 16 | 1 | 1 | 16 |
| | 2 | 16 | 2 | 2 | 16 |
| | 3 | 15 | 3 | 3 | 15 |
| | 4 | 15 | 4 | 4 | 15 |
| | 5 | 14 | 5 | 5 | 14 |
| | 6 | 13 | 6 | 6 | 13 |
| | 7 | 12 | 7 | 7 | 12 |
| | 8 | 12 | 8 | 8 | 12 |
| | 9 | 12 | 9 | 9 | 12 |
| | 10 | 12 | 10 | 10 | 12 |
| | 11 | 12 | 11 | 11 | 12 |
| | 12 | 12 | 12 | 12 | 12 |
| | 13 | 12 | 13 | 13 | 12 |
| | 14 | 12 | 14 | 14 | 12 |
| | 15 | 12 | 15 | 15 | 12 |
| | 16 | 12 | 16 | 16 | 12 |
| Luteal Phase | 17 | **12** | 16.78 | 17 | **12** |
| | 18 | **12** | 17.56 | 18 | **(12+14)/2 = 13** |
| | 19 | **14** | 18.34 | | |
| | 20 | **13** | 19.12 | 19 | **13** |
| | 21 | **13** | 19.9 | 20 | **13** |
| | 22 | **12** | 20.68 | 21 | **(12+16)/2 = 14** |
| | 23 | **16** | 21.46 | | |
| | 24 | **13** | 22.24 | 22 | **13** |
| | 25 | **14** | 23.02 | 23 | **14** |
| | 26 | 15 | 24 | 24 | 15 |
| | 27 | 17 | 25 | 25 | 17 |
| | 28 | 15 | 26 | 26 | 15 |
| | 29 | 16 | 27 | 27 | 16 |
| | 30 | 16 | 28 | 28 | 16 |

**Figure 5.** A worked hypothetical example of continuous standardization for a menstrual cycle greater than 28-days (i.e., 30-day cycle).

## 4. Conclusions

To conclude, this chapter describes two methods to standardize menstrual cycle data, including phasic and continuous standardization. By employing these methods, researchers will be able to more effectively examine fluctuations in addictive behaviors across the menstrual cycle, by allowing data from females with variable cycle lengths to be directly compared or combined across participants. Furthermore, this chapter provides standardization methods which can be used to enhance our understanding of the menstrual cycle as a female-specific factor that may influence important outcome variables in the field of addiction and mental health. Standardized data using continuous standardization also allows for the use of more intricate statistical methods such as TVEM [19] which will significantly benefit behavioral research on the menstrual cycle.

## Acknowledgements

At the time this chapter was written, Ms. Joyce's graduate studies were supported by a Nova Scotia Graduate Scholarship, a Scotia Scholar Award from the Nova Scotia Health Research Foundation, and a Joseph Armand Bombardier Canada Graduate Scholarship from the Social Sciences and Humanities Research Council of Canada (SSHRC). Dr. Stewart is supported through a Canadian Institutes of Health Research (CIHR) Tier 1 Canada Research Chair in Addictions and Mental Health at Dalhousie University.

## Conflict of interest

The authors have no conflicts of interest to declare.

## Author details

Kayla M. Joyce[1] and Sherry H. Stewart[1,2]*

*Address all correspondence to: sstewart@dal.ca

1 Department of Psychiatry, Dalhousie University, Halifax, NS, Canada

2 Department of Psychology and Neuroscience, Dalhousie University, Life Sciences Centre, Halifax, NS, Canada

## References

[1] Stewart SH, Gavric D, Collins P. Women, girls, and alcohol. In: Brady KT, Back SE, Greenfield SF, editors. Women Addict. A Comprehensive Handbook. New York: Guildford Press; 2009. pp. 341-359

[2] National Council on Alcohol and Drug Dependence. Alcoholism, Drug Dependence and Women. 2015. Available from: http://www.ncadd.org/about-addiction/addiction-update/alcoholism-drug-dependence-and-women

[3] Substance Abuse and Mental Health Services Administration. Results from the 2013 National Survey on Drug Use and Health: Summary of National Findings (NIH Publication No. 14-4863). 2014. Available from: https://www.samhsa.gov/data/sites/default/files/NSDUHresultsPDFWHTML2013/Web/NSDUHresults 2013.pdf

[4] White A, Castle I-JP, Chen CM, Shirley M, Roach D, Hingson R. Converging patterns of alcohol use and related outcomes among females and males in the United States, 2002 to 2012. Alcoholism, Clinical and Experimental Research. 2015;**39**:1712-1726

[5] Greenfield TK, Room R. Situational norms for drinking and drunkenness: Trends in the US adult population, 1979-1990. Addiction. 1997;**92**:33-47

[6] Hensel DJ, Fortenberry JD, Harezlak J, Anderson JG, Orr DP. A daily diary analysis of vaginal bleeding and coitus among adolescent women. Journal of Adolescent Health. 2004;**34**:391-394

[7] Spitz CJ, Gold AR, Adams DB. Cognitive and hormonal factors affecting coital frequency. Archives of Sexual Behavior. 1975;**4**:249-263

[8] Steinberg JL, Cherek DR. Menstrual cycle and cigarette smoking behavior. Addictive Behaviors. 1989;**14**:173-179

[9] Mello NK, Mendelson JH, Palmieri SL. Cigarette smoking by women: Interactions with alcohol use. Psychopharmacology. 1987;**93**:8-15

[10] Münster Ki SL, Helm P. Length and variation in the menstrual cycle—A cross-sectional study from a Danish county. Journal of Obstetrics and Gynaecology. 1992;**99**:422-429

[11] Feher J. Female reproductive physiology. In: Feher J, editor. Quantitative Human Physiology. Boston: Abademic Press; 2012. pp. 846-855

[12] Griffin JE, Ojeda SR. Textbook of Endocrine Physiology. New York: Oxford University Press; 2004

[13] Groome NP, Illingworth PJ, O'Brien M, Pai R, Rodger FE, Mather JP, et al. Measurement of dimeric inhibin b throughout the human menstrual cycle. The Journal of Clinical Endocrinology and Metabolism. 1996;**81**:1401-1405

[14] Levy M, Koeppen B, Stanton B. Berne and Levy Principles of Physiology. St. Louis, Missouri: Mosby; 2000

[15] Lenton EA, Landgren BM, Sexton L. Normal variation in the length of the luteal phase of the menstrual cycle: Indentification of the short luteal phase. British Journal of Obstetrics and Gynaecology. 1984;**91**:685-689

[16] Fehring RJ, Schneider M, Raviele K. Variability in the phases of the menstrual cycle. Journal of Obstetric, Gynecologic, and Neonatal Nursing. 2006;**35**:376-384

[17] Walsh RN, Budtz-Olsen I, Leader C, Cummins RA. The menstrual cycle, personality, and academic performance. Archives of General Psychiatry. 1981;**38**:219-221

[18] Tan X, Shiyko MP, Li R, Li Y, Dierker L. A time-varying effect model for intensive longitudinal data. Psychological Methods. 2012;**17**:61-77

[19] Joyce KM, Hudson A, O'Connor R, Thompson K, Hodgin M, Perrot T, et al. Changes in coping and social motives for drinking and alcohol consumption across the menstrual cycle. Depression and Anxiety. 2018;**35**(4):313-320